Francy Brethenoux-Seguin et Denis Lenoble

Communiquer en anglais

Santé et soins

6e édition

Vuibert

Francy Brethenoux-Seguin est professeur d'anglais. Elle dispense des formations en IFSI et à l'Institut européen de formation en santé Paris.

Denis Lenoble est cadre de santé et formateur en IFSI.

L'autrice remercie Susanne Spencer, Françoise Digel et Caroline Williams. Elle remercie également Lisa Dial (aide-soignante en soins palliatifs à Paris) pour sa participation à la rédaction de l'unité 13.

L'éditeur remercie chaleureusement Adrien Hermans et Frédéric Devanlay du studio BigWheels pour l'enregistrement audio et la direction des voix anglaises, ainsi que les deux comédiens, Kim Tilbury et Saul Jephcott.

Couverture : Primo & Primo
Maquette et mise en pages : CB Defretin
Illustrations :
© A.C.R. : Anne-Christel Rolling
© C.K. : Caroline Koehly
© S.M. : Sandrine Marchand
© Magnard

ISBN : 978-2-311-66204-7

Avant-propos

Un outil de formation à l'anglais professionnel infirmier

L'anglais étant une unité d'enseignement (UE) obligatoire de la formation en soins infirmiers, nous avons souhaité proposer aux étudiants et à leurs enseignants une méthode spécifique d'apprentissage de la langue. Cet outil a pour but de permettre aux élèves de « communiquer en anglais dans le domaine de la santé et des soins et d'acquérir du vocabulaire professionnel » comme l'exigent les objectifs des semestres 1, 2 et 3 de l'UE 6.2.

Ces objectifs sont traités à travers 13 unités au cours desquelles les apprenants vont suivre l'itinéraire d'un patient anglophone : son arrivée aux urgences, son séjour à l'hôpital, puis son retour à domicile ou sa prise en charge en soins palliatifs. Il suit une progression qui permet de revenir sur les bases de la langue tout en appréhendant les situations professionnelles les plus fréquentes.

Une méthode pédagogique pour faciliter l'apprentissage et la pratique de la langue

Chaque unité est constituée d'outils pédagogiques variés facilitant l'apprentissage de la langue dans le contexte propre à la santé et aux soins. Vous retrouverez :

- des **dialogues illustrant des situations professionnelles courantes** à télécharger. Il sont destinés à faire l'objet d'une étude guidée ;

Téléchargez les pistes audio à l'adresse suivante
https://www.vuibert.fr/site/662047

- des exercices permettant de travailler :
  - **la compréhension orale** avec des questions portant sur les dialogues et des exercices d'écoute (également disponibles en téléchargement),
  - **l'expression orale** avec des jeux de rôle et des sujets de débats,
  - **l'expression et la compréhension écrites** avec des exercices en contexte.
  - Pour chaque unité, retrouvez **2 exercices interactifs à faire** en ligne pour s'auto-évaluer !
- des **encadrés grammaticaux synthétiques**, assortis d'exercices d'application afin de percevoir et mémoriser d'une façon simple les principales règles de la langue anglaise ;
- une aide à la compréhension, à l'acquisition et à la **mémorisation du vocabulaire professionnel** :
  - sous la forme d'encadrés et de schémas,
  - avec des **schémas anatomiques en couleurs** pour réviser le vocabulaire des principaux systèmes anatomiques.

L'intégralité des schémas, dans leurs versions vierges et corrigées, est accessible en téléchargement à l'aide des liens et QR codes tout au long du livre.

Un ouvrage pour accompagner des projets professionnels

Au-delà de l'apprentissage de la langue dans le contexte du programme des études, cet ouvrage pourra être utile aux professionnels de la santé qui désirent acquérir une meilleure maîtrise de la langue anglaise afin d'améliorer leur relation avec les patients anglophones. Il s'adresse également à ceux qui ont le projet de partir dans un pays où l'anglais est la langue privilégiée, ou à ceux qui désirent travailler dans l'humanitaire et le développement.

Contents

UNIT 1

UNIT 1 Admitting a patient to the accident and emergency department

Toutes les pistes audio de l'unité à télécharger ici
https://www.lienmini.fr/angsoinu1

Piste 1 Dialogue between Mr Brown and the nurse

Traduction p. 204

Listen to the dialogue. Mr Brown is being admitted to hospital.

Mr Brown Good afternoon. I've hurt myself. Can you help me, please?
Nurse Certainly. Do you speak French?
Mr Brown No, not at all. I'm sorry.
Nurse What happened?
Mr Brown I fell off a ladder.
Nurse Where does it hurt?
Mr Brown My leg hurts*. I think it is broken.
Nurse *(talking to another nurse)*
Can you bring an air splint*, please?
(talking to Mr Brown)
Don't worry. Everything will be all right.
Can you lie on the trolley*, please?

In the emergency cubicle*.

Nurse Are you allergic to* any medicines, aspirin for instance?
Mr Brown No, I'm not. But I'm allergic to iodine and penicillin.
Nurse I'm going to give you a painkiller by intravenous* injection.
You are attached to a monitor so I can read your heartbeat*.
Mr Brown I take medication for my blood pressure*.
Nurse Do you take any other drugs?
Mr Brown Yes, I do, but I don't remember their names.
I'm diabetic and I have angina*.
Nurse Have you ever had an operation?
Mr Brown Yes, I have. For my gall bladder*,
five years ago.
Nurse Do you smoke?
Mr Brown Yes, I smoke about twenty cigarettes a day.

To help you

- **I'm hurt:** je suis blessé
- **my leg hurts:** j'ai mal à la jambe
- **air splint:** attelle gonflable/à dépression
- **trolley:** brancard
- **emergency cubicle:** box des urgences
- **to be allergic to:** être allergique à
- **intravenous (IV):** intraveineuse
- **heartbeat:** rythme cardiaque
- **blood pressure:** tension artérielle
- **angina:** angine de poitrine
- **gall bladder:** vésicule biliaire

Questions sur le dialogue

1. Does Mr Brown speak good French? ....

2. What happened to him? ....

3. Where does it hurt? ....

4. What does the nurse need to carry Mr Brown to the emergency cubicle? ....

5. What is Mr Brown allergic to? ....

6. Does he smoke a lot? ....

GRAMMAR

Present simple

• Emploi

On utilise le présent simple pour décrire des actes routiniers, habituels ou des situations permanentes.
Il peut être accompagné des adverbes de fréquence : *always, never, often, sometimes, usually,* etc.
Il prend un "s" à la 3e personne du singulier : he works.

• Construction

Forme affirmative	Sujet + verbe	They work in this hospital. She works in this hospital.
Forme négative	Sujet + do not (don't)/does not (doesn't) + verbe	We don't speak English. He doesn't speak English.
Forme interrogative	Auxiliaire do/does + sujet + verbe	Do you smoke? – Yes, I do. – No, I don't. Does he smoke? – Yes, he does. – No, he doesn't.

Travaillez à deux : Révisez le présent simple

Posez ces questions à votre partenaire, inscrivez ses réponses ; puis inversez les rôles.

How are you? : ....

Where do you come from? : ....

Where do you live? : ....

Is it far from the hospital? : ....

Are you married? : ....

Do you have/Have you got any children? : ....

What are their names? : ....

How old are you? : ....

How tall are you? : ....

What is your weight? : ....

What do you do? What's your job?/What is your occupation? : ....

Do you like your job? : ....

What time do you get up in the morning? : ....

What time do you usually start work? : ....

To help you

- **once a week:** une fois par semaine
- **twice a month:** deux fois par mois
- **five times a year:** cinq fois par an

GRAMMAR

Comment poser une question ?

• Emploi

Deux possibilités :
– question fermée, avec réponses attendue par oui/non ;
– question ouverte, avec réponse précise.

• Construction

1. Questions (yes/no questions)

Réponse avec un seul mot :
– What's your name? Fanny.

Auxiliaire du temps utilisé	Sujet	Verbe
Do	you	take medication for your heart?
Have	they	worked in this unit before?
Could	you	spell your name?

2. Questions ouvertes

Les réponses attendues sont précises et construites.
– How do you feel today?

3. Questions avec mots interrogatifs

Les mots interrogatifs les plus courants sont :

Mot interrogatif	Renseignement que l'on désire obtenir	Exemple
What…?	Qu'est ce qui… ?	What does his x-ray show?
Who…?	Qui… ?	Who is giving this injection?
When…?	Quand… ?	When is the surgery planned?
Where…?	Où… ?	Where does it hurt?
Why…?	Pourquoi… ?	Why did you say that?
Which…?	Lequel… ?	Which treatment do you prefer?
How…?	Comment… ?	How do you spell that?
How many (+ pluriel)…?	Combien… ?	How many patients are there in the ward?
How much (+ singulier)…?	Combien… ?	How much do you weigh?

Exercice 1

Réponse p. 14

Posez les questions commençant par how afin d'obtenir les réponses écrites en bleu.

1. She is **1 metre 70.** ……………………………………
2. **Twenty** nurses work on this ward. ……………………………………
3. This new stethoscope is expensive. It is **90 Euros**. ……………………………………
4. He is **32**. ……………………………………
5. The operating theatre is **half a mile away**. ……………………………………

Exercice 2

Réponse p. 14

Vous désirez obtenir des renseignements supplémentaires concernant un patient, posez-lui ces questions en anglais :

1. Combien mesurez-vous ? : ....
2. Combien pesez-vous ? : ....
3. Combien de litres d'eau buvez-vous par jour ? : ....

Trouvez les réponses du patient en utilisant les données ci-dessous.

- 1 inch (in) = 2,54 cm
- 1 foot (ft) = 30 cm
- 1 ounce (oz) = 28 g
- 1 pound (lb) = 450 g
- 1 stone (st) = 6,3 kg
- 1,7 pints (pt) = 1 litre

1. ....
2. ....
3. ....

Exercice 3

Réponse p. 14

Reliez la question à la réponse qui lui correspond.

1. What does he like? ....
2. How is he? ....
3. What is he like? ....
4. What does he look like? .... (physical appearance)

...... **A.** Not very well today. He has a cold.
...... **B.** He is quite small, with blond hair.
...... **C.** He likes playing cards.
...... **D.** He's very open and friendly.

Exercice 4

Réponse p. 14

Posez les questions afin d'obtenir les réponses écrites en bleu.

Ex.: This year, I'm going to **Ireland** on holiday. = *Where are you going on holiday this year?*

1. Mr Brown is going to visit **friends**. ....
2. He'll need to take a lot of **medication** with him. ....
3. Hurry up! **The intern** is about to leave. ....
4. He'll have a **stroke** if he keeps on smoking. ....
5. He's going to spend a week **in this unit**. ....

Piste 2

Exercice 5 : Filling in an admission form

Traduction pp. 204-205
Réponse p. 14

Écoutez le dialogue et complétez la conversation entre la réceptionniste et Mme Brown. Utilisez les phrases suivantes :

- What is his surname?
- Have you got social security cover*
- Where was he born?
- Where are you staying…
- What is the name of your GP*?
- Could you spell it, please?
- And his first name?
- What is your phone number in France?

Receptionist Excuse me, could you give me some information about your husband please. I need to fill in his admission form.
(1) ....

Mrs Brown Brown.

Receptionist (2) ....

Mrs Brown B.R.O.W.N.

Receptionist (3) ....

Mrs Brown James.

Receptionist (4) ....

Mrs Brown In Bath, in England.

Receptionist Now, I need more information about your address. (5) .... at the moment, please?

Mrs Brown We're staying in Ruffec, 21 rue Aunay.

Receptionist What is your home address?

Mrs Brown 12, Raven Street, Bath, England.

Receptionist Could you speak more slowly, please? Thank you. (6) ....

Mrs Brown 05 45 12 43 76.

Receptionist (7) ....?
All right. Could you give me your insurance form and your European card, please?

Mrs Brown Here they are.

Receptionist Thank you (8) ....?

Mrs Brown Doctor Daniels, 12, London Street, Bath.

To help you

- **social security cover:** assurance maladie (se dit aussi medical insurance)
- **GP (general practitioner):** médecin traitant

Piste 3

Exercice 6 : L'alphabet

Réponse p. 14

Écoutez, puis répétez.

A	E	I	O	U	G	H	J
K	P	Q	R	W	X	Y	Z

Écoutez, puis soulignez les lettres que vous entendez.

B F K A C Y I

Travaillez à deux : Remplir une fiche d'admission

Posez les questions à votre partenaire afin de remplir la fiche d'admission ci-dessous.

Surname/Family name (Mr/Mrs/Miss) ....

First name ....

Date of birth ....

Place of birth ....

Marital status ....

Temporary address in France ....

....

Permanent address ....

....

Name and address of next of kin[1] ....

....

Name and address of GP ....

....

Current occupation ....

....

....

1 Next of kin : parent proche, sous-entendu la personne à prévenir.

Piste 4 Exercice 7

Réponse p. 14

Écoutez, puis répétez les mots se référant à la chambre d'un patient.

- locker
- towel
- washcloth
- comb
- brush
- gown
- cup
- napkin
- drawer
- bedside table
- washbasin
- folding screen
- wheelchair
- armchair
- blanket
- pillow
- curtain
- call button/ call bell

A patient's room

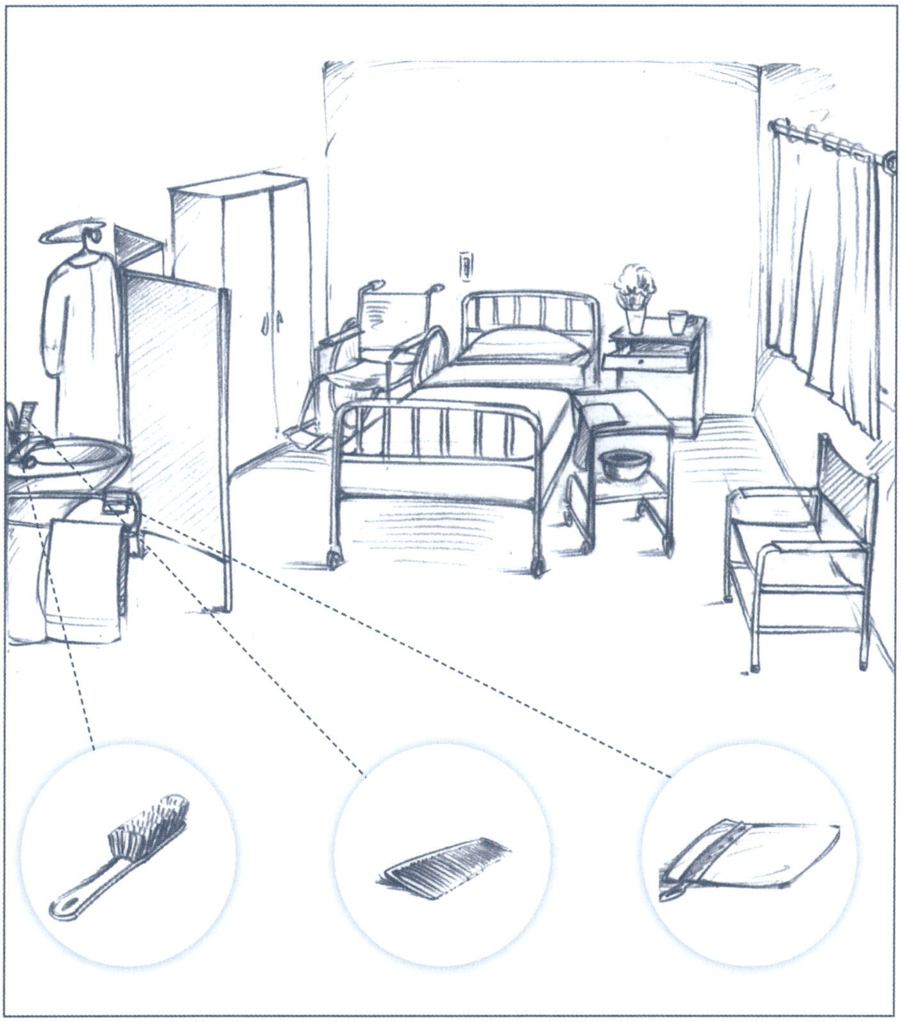

© C.K.

https://www.lienmini.fr/angsoin02

Écrivez les équivalents français désignant les objets présents sur le dessin.

- **1.** locker: ....
- **2.** towel: ....
- **3.** washcloth: ....
- **4.** comb: ....
- **5.** brush: ....
- **6.** gown: ....
- **7.** cup: ....
- **8.** napkin: ....
- **9.** drawer: ....
- **10.** bedside table: ....
- **11.** washbasin: ....
- **12.** folding screen: ....
- **13.** wheelchair: ....
- **14.** armchair: ....
- **15.** blanket: ....
- **16.** pillow: ....
- **17.** curtain: ....
- **18.** call button/call bell: .....
- **19.** sheet: ....
- **20.** sick bowl: ....
- **21.** trolley: ....

Piste 5 — Exercice 8

Réponse p. 14

Écoutez, puis répétez.
Dans la liste ci-dessous, les mots font référence aux besoins fondamentaux. Regroupez-les par thèmes.

- to breathe
- psychological need
- to eat
- to eliminate
- to drink
- cultural need
- spiritual need
- to move about
- social need
- to maintain a normal body temperature

Physical needs	Other needs

Piste 6 — Exercice 9

Réponse p. 15

Écoutez, puis répétez.
Complétez la légende à l'aide des mots suivants :

- tooth/teeth
- tongue
- chin
- hair
- ear
- nose
- cheek
- eyebrow
- eye
- lip
- mouth
- forehead

The face

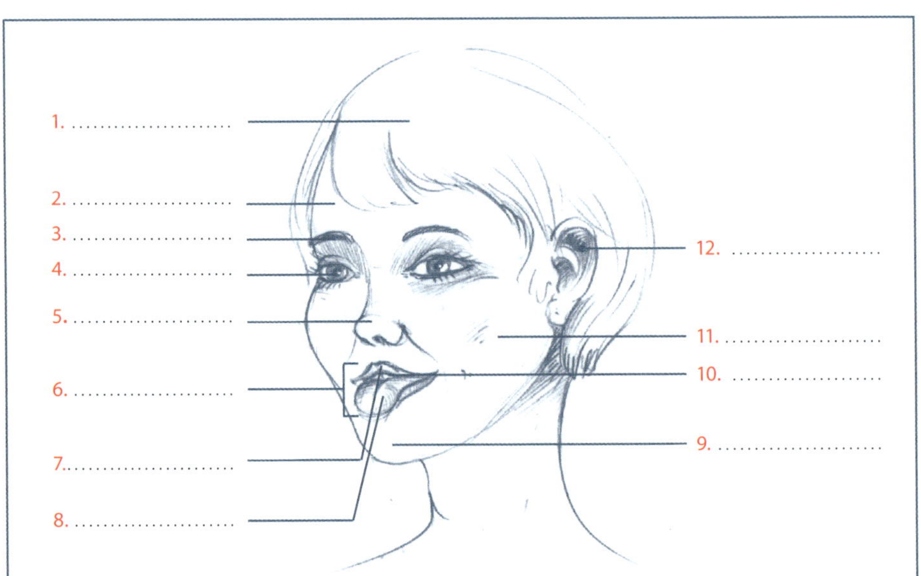

https://www.lienmini.fr/angsoin03

Travaillez à deux : Stress

Posez à votre partenaire la question ci-dessous puis inversez les rôles. Répondez en donnant des exemples précis.

Why do these situations sometimes cause stress?

- the change of pace in contemporary life
- when something has to be done quickly at work without explanation
- any major life change such as: relationship break-up/divorce
- miscarriage, abortion
- adjusting to another culture
- unemployment
- a serious or debilitating illness such as cancer
- invasive surgery
- abuse (physical/psychological/emotional)
- feeling isolated

Exercice 10 : Testez-vous !

Réponse p. 15

Traduisez en anglais.

1. Où avez-vous mal ? ....

2. Où souffrez-vous ? ....

3. Mes yeux me font mal. ....

4. Que fait-elle ? Elle est infirmière. ....

5. Il est allergique aux antibiotiques. ....

6. Tous les combien prenez-vous ces médicaments ? : ....

7. Combien de cigarettes fumez-vous par jour ? : ....

Exercice 11 : Patient information

Réponse p. 15

Welcome to the accident & emergency department

Cochez la (les) bonne(s) affirmation(s).

	True	False
1. First you will be registered at the reception desk and then the triage nurse* will assess* the seriousness of your complaint*, and determine the degree of urgency.		
2. Based on the seriousness of your condition*, you will be assigned* a degree of urgency.		
3. Patients are not treated in order of arrival, but rather according to the degree of urgency.		
4. After the emergency physician has examined you, tests such as blood tests, ECG, urine tests or x-rays will be done if necessary. You may need to wait a few hours for those results.		
5. As soon as the diagnosis and first treatment at accident & emergency are finished, we will take you to your room as soon as possible.		

To help you

- **triage nurse:** infirmière régulatrice
- **to assess:** évaluer
- **complaint:** maladie, affection
- **condition:** état
- **to assign:** attribuer

https://www.lienmini.fr/angsoinq1a

Vocabulary quiz: Patient's room

Réponse p. 15

Complétez chaque définition avec le terme correct.

1. A large cover used on beds to keep people warm is called a ....
a) sheet **b)** gown **c)** blanket **d)** coat

2. A .... is used for any type of nausea.
a) washbasin **b)** drawer **c)** sick bowl **d)** bedside table

3. To make a bed you need two white ....
a) pillows **b)** sheets **c)** curtains **d)** blankets

4. A .... is used to rest* your head on in bed.
a) curtain **b)** clothe **c)** napkin **d)** pillow

5. A piece of clothing worn* in a hospital by someone doing or having an operation is a ....
a) blanket **b)** sheet **c)** gown **d)** pyjama

https://www.lienmini.fr/angsoinq1b

Anatomy quiz: The face

Réponse p. 15

Complétez chaque affirmation avec le terme correct.

1. The .... is in the mouth and used for tasting, swallowing* and speaking.
a) nose **b)** lip **c)** chin **d)** tongue

2. The .... is either side of the face below the eyes.
a) ear **b)** cheek
c) forehead **d)** mouth

3. The .... grows especially on the head.
a) eyebrow **b)** tongue
c) hair **d)** face

4. The .... is used for breathing* and smelling things.
a) eye **b)** ear
c) nose **d)** lip

5. The .... is either of the two edges* at the opening* of the mouth.
a) lip **b)** cheek **c)** eye **d)** tooth

To help you

- **to rest:** reposer
- **wear, wore, worn:** porter (vêtement)
- **to swallow:** avaler
- **to breath:** respirer
- **edge:** bord
- **opening:** entrée, ouverture

Medical Vocabulary: unit 1

- **illness:** maladie
- **needs:** besoins
- **sick:** malade
- **painkiller:** calmant
- **heartbeat:** rythme cardiaque
- **blood pressure:** pression artérielle
- **to breathe:** respirer
- **headache:** mal de tête
- **to weigh:** peser
- **angina:** angine de poitrine
- **intravenous:** intraveineuse

Let's discuss!

Admitting a patient at the Accident and Emergency department

Mr Brown arrives at the Emergency department with his wife. He is doubled up with pain.

What are you going to do? What are the essential steps in the procedure for admitting this patient and welcoming his wife?
What improvements would you suggest for the admission of patients into hospital?

Corrigés

Exercice 1

1. How tall is she?
2. How many nurses work on this ward?
3. How much is it?
4. How old is he?
5. How far is the operating theatre?

Exercice 2

1. How tall are you?
2. How much do you weigh?
3. How many litres of water do you drink per/a day?

Exercice 3

1. C 2. A 3. D 4. B

Exercice 4

1. Who is Mr Brown going to visit?
2. What will he need to take with him?
3. Who is about to leave?
4. What will he have if he keeps on smoking?
5. Where is he going to spend a week?

Exercice 5

1. What is his surname?
2. Could you spell it, please?
3. And his first name?
4. Where was he born?
5. Where are you staying...
6. What is your phone number in France?
7. Have you got social security cover ?
8. What is the name of your GP?

Exercice 6

K – A – Y – I

Exercice 7

1. locker: placard
2. towel: serviette de toilette
3. washcloth: gant de toilette
4. comb: peigne
5. brush: brosse
6. gown: chemise de nuit
7. cup: tasse
8. napkin: serviette de table
9. drawer: tiroir
10. bedside table: table de nuit
11. washbasin: lavabo
12. folding screen: paravent
13. wheelchair: fauteuil roulant
14. armchair: fauteuil
15. blanket: couverture
16. pillow: oreiller
17. curtain: rideau
18. call button/call bell: sonnette
19. sheet: drap
20. sick bowl: haricot
21. trolley: chariot

Exercice 8

Physical needs	Other needs
to breathe to eat to eliminate to drink to move about to maintain a normal body temperature	psychological need cultural need spiritual need social need

Corrigés

Exercice 9

1. hair
2. forehead
3. eyebrow
4. eye
5. nose
6. mouth
7. lip
8. tongue
9. chin
10. tooth/teeth
11. cheek
12. ear

Exercice 10 : Testez-vous !

1. Where does it hurt?
2. Where is the pain?
3. My eyes hurt/I have got a pain in my eyes.
4. What does she do? She is a nurse.
5. He is allergic to antibiotics.
6. How often do you take these medicines/drugs?
7. How many cigarettes do you smoke a/per day?

Exercice 11

1. True
2. True
3. True
4. True
5. True

Vocabulary quiz: Patient's room

1. blanket
2. sick bowl
3. sheets
4. pillow
5. gown

Anatomy quiz: The face

1. tongue
2. cheek
3. hair
4. nose
5. lip

UNIT 2

UNIT 2

Asking for directions

Toutes les pistes audio de l'unité à télécharger ici
https://www.lienmini.fr/angsoinu2

Piste 7

Dialogue between Mike and a woman in the street, and Mike and the receptionist

Traduction p. 205

Listen to the dialogue. Mr Brown's son, Mike, is on his way to the hospital to visit his father.

Mike	Excuse me. Could you tell me the way to the hospital, please?
Woman	Certainly. It's on the corner of the main street. Go straight on, then turn right before the roundabout*.
Mike	Is it after the traffic lights?
Woman	Yes, opposite the chemist's*, next to the post office.
Mike	How far is it exactly?
Woman	About a ten-minute walk.
Mike	Thank you very much.
Woman	Not at all.

A few minutes later, at the hospital reception desk.

Mike	I'd like to visit Mr Brown. Could you tell me where his room is, please?
Receptionist	Yes, it's on the medical ward*.
Mike	Which floor* is it on?
Receptionist	It's on the third floor.
Mike	Is there a lift*?
Receptionist	Yes, at the end of the corridor. Take the lift to the third floor. As you get out of the lift, turn left and go down the corridor. It's the first door on your left.
Mike	Thank you.
Receptionist	You're welcome.

To help you

- **roundabout:** rond-point
- **chemist's** (GB): pharmacie
- **ward:** service
- **floor:** étage
- **lift** (GB), **elevator** (US): ascenseur

Questions sur le dialogue

1. Who is Mike? ....
2. Why does he want to go to the hospital? ....
3. Where is it? ....
4. Is it far away? ....
5. On which ward is his father's room? ....
6. Which floor is it on? ....

GRAMMAR

La date

Comment dire la date	Comment écrire la date
• *The* et *of* ne s'écrivent pas mais se prononcent. – Ex.: (The) nineteenth (of) January. • On emploie l'adjectif numéral (ex: fifth). • Le millésime se divise en deux : 1999 (nineteen ninety-nine).	• Manière la plus courante : 14 August 2010. • Autres possibilités : - 14th August 2010 - August 14(th) 2010 - 14.8.10. • On met toujours une majuscule au mois.

Piste 8

Exercice 1

Écoutez, puis répétez.

- 1st: the first
- 2nd: the second
- 3rd: the third
- 4th: the fourth
- 5th: the fifth
- 6th: the sixth
- 8th: the eighth
- 9th: the ninth
- 20th: the twentieth

Exercice 2

Réponse p. 31

Dans le dialogue page 18, soulignez les expressions concernant les directions. Puis traduisez la liste ci-dessous.

1. Allez tout droit : ....
2. Tournez à gauche : ....
3. Au bout du couloir : ....
4. Près de : ....
5. Sur votre droite : ....
6. En face de : ....
7. Au troisième étage : ....

GRAMMAR

Present continuous

• Emploi

a) On utilise le present continuous pour parler de choses qui sont en train de se passer maintenant, lorsque l'action se déroule au moment où l'on parle.
On utilise les expressions de temps telles que : now, at the moment, etc.
– He is working at the moment.

b) On utilise également le present continuous pour évoquer des projets proches dans le temps.
On utilise les expressions de temps telles que : tomorrow, next week, in three hours, at five o'clock, today, etc.
– What are you doing this weekend?
– I am going to the cinema with friends.

• Construction

Forme affirmative	Sujet + auxiliaire + verbe à la forme -ing	I am reading a medical magazine now.
Forme négative	Sujet + auxiliaire à la forme négative + verbe à la forme -ing	She is not (isn't) reading a medical magazine at the moment.
Forme interrogative	Auxiliaire + sujet + verbe à la forme -ing	Are you reading a medical magazine?

• Remarques

– Exceptions : les verbes exprimant un sentiment ou une pensée n'ont pas de forme progressive.
Ex.: dislike, hate, like, love, want, know, believe, etc.
– Lorsqu'on emploie always avec le present continuous, il se traduit alors par : sans arrêt, constamment, tout le temps : She is always meeting interesting people in this department.

Exercice 3

Réponse p. 31

Passez du présent simple au présent progressif en effectuant les changements nécessaires.

Ex.: What do you usually do **at weekends**? What are you doing **this weekend**?

1. Do you visit him on the geriatric ward every week? .... this week?
2. Does the surgeon operate every Friday? .... next Friday?
3. Do you come to this hospital? .... next month?
4. Does she work in this unit? .... at the moment?
5. What does this patient have for lunch? .... today?

Exercice 4

Réponse p. 31

Complétez ce dialogue en utilisant le présent simple ou le présent progressif (continu).

Nurse What **(1)** .... (*you / do*)?

Patient I **(2)** .... (*pack*) my case. I **(3)** .... (*leave*).

Nurse But I **(4)** .... (*not / understand*). Why **(5)** .... (*you / leave*)?

Patient I can't stand being in hospital. I **(6)** .... (*not / want*) to have an operation.

Nurse But you can't! Where **(7)** .... (*you / go*)?

Patient My girlfriend **(8)** .... (*wait for*) me. We **(9)** .... (go) home.

GRAMMAR

Prépositions de lieu et de mouvement

• Prépositions de lieu

On utilise les prépositions suivantes pour décrire où se trouve quelqu'un ou quelque chose.

- in: dans
- on: sur
- on top of: en haut de
- at the top & bottom: en haut & en bas, au fond
- inside & outside: à l'intérieur & à l'extérieur
- near: près de
- next to: à côté de
- in front of: devant
- behind: derrière
- opposite: en face de
- under: sous, au-dessous de
- over: au-dessus de
- at: à
- on the left/right (of): à gauche/ à droite (de)
- among: parmi
- between: entre

• Prépositions de mouvement

On utilise les prépositions suivantes pour décrire un mouvement.
Elles sont le plus souvent employées avec des verbes tel que : bring, carry, go, come, walk, run, take, get, push.

- along: le long de
- up: en haut
- down: en bas
- into: dans (sens dynamique)
- out of: hors de
- away: loin
- from: de (indique la provenance)
- to: à, vers (implique un déplacement)
- through: à travers (trois dimensions)
- across: de l'autre côté, à travers (deux dimensions)
- past: devant (implique un mouvement)
- around: autour

Exercice 5

Réponse p. 31

Reliez le verbe à la traduction qui lui correspond.

1. to bring somebody **along** .... •	• .... **A.** descendre
2. to come **up to** .... •	• .... **B.** venir/monter à
3. to go **down** .... •	• .... **C.** amener quelqu'un avec soi
4. to run **into** .... •	• .... **D.** partir en courant
5. to get **out of** bed .... •	• .... **E.** rentrer dans (collision)
6. to run **away** .... •	• .... **F.** venir de
7. to come **from** .... •	• .... **G.** se lever

8. to go **to** .... •	• .... **H.** emmener (une personne)
9. to push **through** .... •	• .... **I.** traverser en courant
10. to run **across** .... •	• .... **J.** aller à
11. to take **along** .... •	• .... **K.** se frayer, s'ouvrir un chemin
12. to walk **around** .... •	• .... **L.** tourner à gauche/à droite
13. to turn **left/right** .... •	• .... **M.** faire le tour

Exercice 6

Réponse p. 31

Complétez les phrases suivantes en utilisant les prépositions de lieu indiquées entre parenthèses.

1. There is a disabled person .... us (*parmi*). Could you be kind and help her, please?
2. The pharmacy is .... the operating room (*en face de*).
3. The bus stop is .... the entrance of the hospital (*devant*).
4. Mrs Parker is getting .... the taxi (*dans*).
5. I was working .... the 8th floor of the hospital (*au*).
6. The walkway is .... this building (*derrière*).
7. Have you looked .... the bed (*sous*)?
8. He sat.................. me (*à côté de*).
9. I'm looking .... the window (*par*).
10. Please lie down .... the bed (*sur*).
11. Now I can walk .... the corridor (*le long*).
12. You can sit .... these two patients (*entre*)

Exercice 7

Réponse p. 31

Choisissez pour chaque phrase la bonne préposition dans la liste ci-dessous.

• below	• above	• behind	• next to	• along	• opposite

1. The water came .... their knees (*au-dessus de*).
2. There is a clinic .... our house (*en face de*).
3. There were ambulances .... the road (*le long de*).
4. I can't see him, he is standing .... the wall (*derrière*).
5. The room .... is free (*au-dessous*).
6. Please, come and sit down .... me (*près de*).

Piste 9

Exercice 8 : A telephone call

Traduction p. 206
Réponse p. 32

Écoutez le dialogue et complétez la conversation entre la réceptionniste et la personne qui appelle. Utilisez les phrases suivantes :

• The line's busy.	• … to call me back as soon as possible	• Who's calling, please?
• How can I help you?	• I'll pass on your message.	

Receptionist Good afternoon. This is the medical ward.
(1) ....

Caller Can I speak to the consultant* or the senior nurse* in charge of Mr Newton, please?

Receptionist **(2)** ....

Caller This is Dr Roberts.

Receptionist I'm sorry, but he isn't in today and the senior nurse is at a meeting.
I'll put you through to one of his secretaries. Hold the line, please. I'm awfully sorry.
(3) ....

Caller Can I leave a message?

Receptionist Yes, certainly.

Caller Could you tell her **(4)** ....

Receptionist Could I have your name again?

Caller Doctor Roberts from Paris and my phone number is 0.1.4.7.5.8.5.8, double 9.

Receptionist All right Doctor Roberts.
(5) ....

Caller Good bye.

To help you

- **consultant:** médecin-chef
- **senior nurse:** cadre de santé

Hospital floor plan

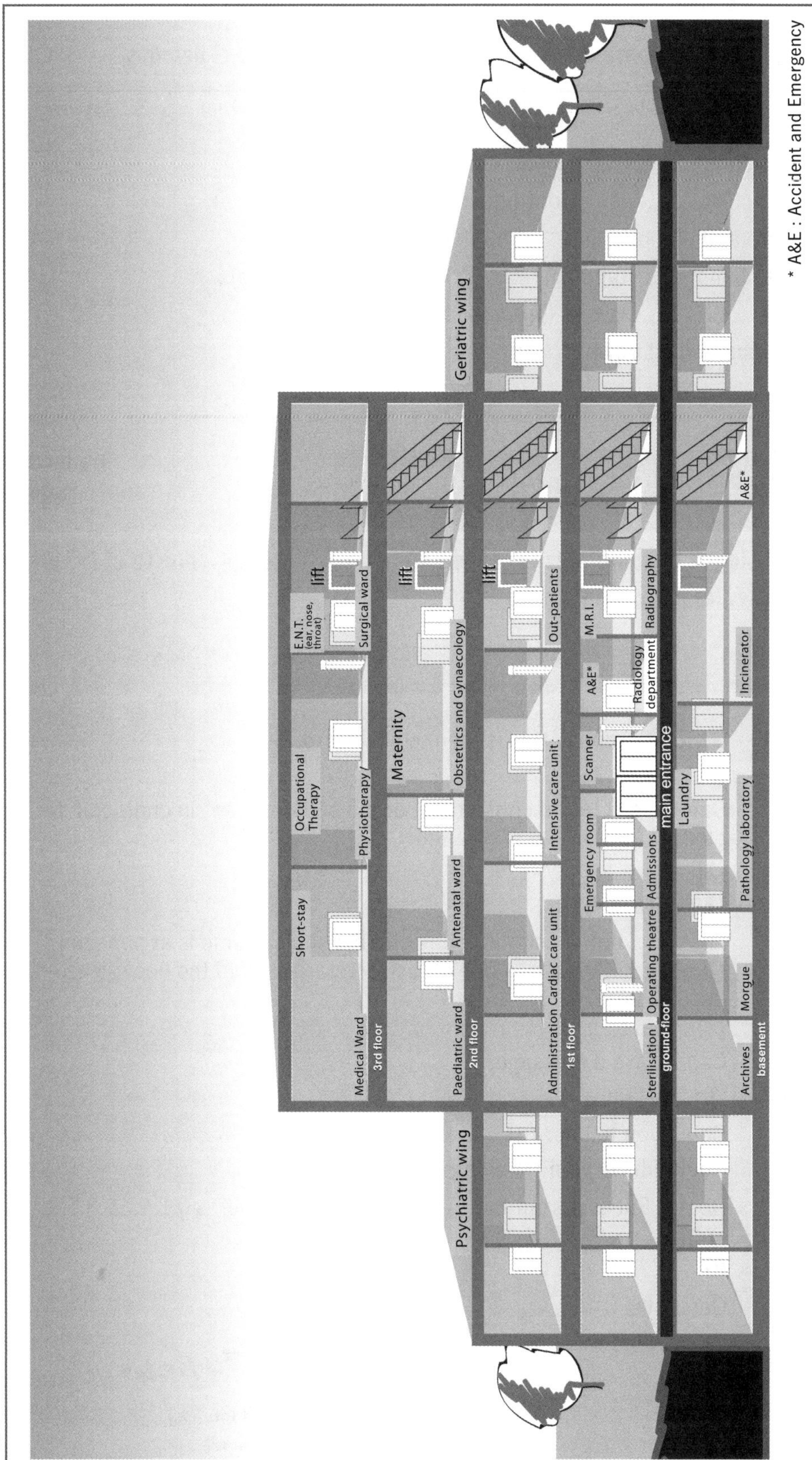

Exercice 9

Réponse p. 32

Observez attentivement le plan de l'hôpital page 24.
Lisez les directions ci-dessous, puis écrivez le nom du service où se trouve le patient.

1. Take the lift to the second floor, follow the corridor, it's the second door on your left.
   The patient is on the ....
2. Take the lift to the third floor, as you get out of the lift, turn right, it's the first door on your right. *The patient is on the* ....
3. It's on the ground floor. Turn right at the main entrance, it's opposite M.R.I.
   The patient is on the ....

Exercice 10

Réponse p. 32

Vous vous trouvez maintenant aux admissions, au rez-de-chaussée (voir plan p. 24). Indiquez à un visiteur les directions à prendre pour se rendre dans les services suivants :

1. The intensive care unit. ....
2. The surgical ward. ....
3. The physiotherapy department. ....

Travaillez à deux : Asking for help

A a besoin de renseignements que B peut lui transmettre. Établissez un dialogue compte tenu des informations ci-dessous.

A. You are from Dublin and have just arrived at the hospital for the first time. You need help.

Situation 1. You have an appointment with Doctor Lavau, but you don't know where his department is.

Situation 2. You need to fill in a form but you don't understand it.

Situation 3. You want to visit a friend, who had an operation yesterday, but you don't know the number and the floor of his/her room.

B. You work in the hospital and know it quite well. You see someone who you think needs help. Look at the information above and try to help him/her.

Situation 1. Dr Lavau works in the cardiac care unit.

Situation 2. See Unit 1. Fillling in an admission form (*p. 7*).

Situation 3. The number of his/her room is 204, it's on the second floor.

Travaillez à deux

A. est une réceptionniste.
B. veut parler à un patient hospitalisé.

Suivez les instructions suivantes (A et B), puis remplissez le bloc-notes (A) :

A. Answer the phone.
B. Ask to speak to Mr Johnson.
A. You don't know Mr Johnson.
B. You apologize and try again.
A. Answer the phone.
B. Ask to speak to Mr Evans.
A. Mr Evans' line is busy. Suggest B to call back.
B. You can't call back. Leave a message.
A. Take the message and fill in the message pad.

Date:
Time:
Message for:
Message:
Caller's name:
Phone number:
Caller will phone back:
Please call back:

Improvisez un autre dialogue téléphonique.

GRAMMAR

Phrase négative

• Formes régulières avec not

La phrase négative est formée avec l'auxiliaire + la marque de la négation (not) :
- She is not (isn't) a nursing auxiliary.
- He will not (won't) call me back.

• Avec no, never, nobody, neither, nor, etc.

Dans une phrase anglaise, on n'emploie jamais deux négations :
- Nobody knows them.
- He never takes his medicine.

• L'impératif négatif

L'impératif négatif est formé du verbe à l'infinitif sans "to" précédé de l'auxiliaire à la forme négative :
- Don't smoke in your room.

Exercice 11

Réponse p. 32

Mettez à la forme négative les phrases suivantes.

1. She is in charge of the cardiac care unit: ....
2. He works in the psychiatric wing: ....
3. They always ring the bell: ....
4. The nursing auxiliary is on duty tonight: ....
5. Run in the corridor: ....

Piste 10 — Exercice 12

Réponse p. 32

Écoutez, puis répétez.
Sur le dessin du corps humain ci-dessous, inscrivez près de chaque chiffre le mot qui lui correspond.

- brain
- small intestine
- heart
- foot/feet
- leg
- diaphragm
- hand
- liver
- thigh
- windpipe/trachea
- stomach
- lung
- forearm
- upper arm
- colon

The body

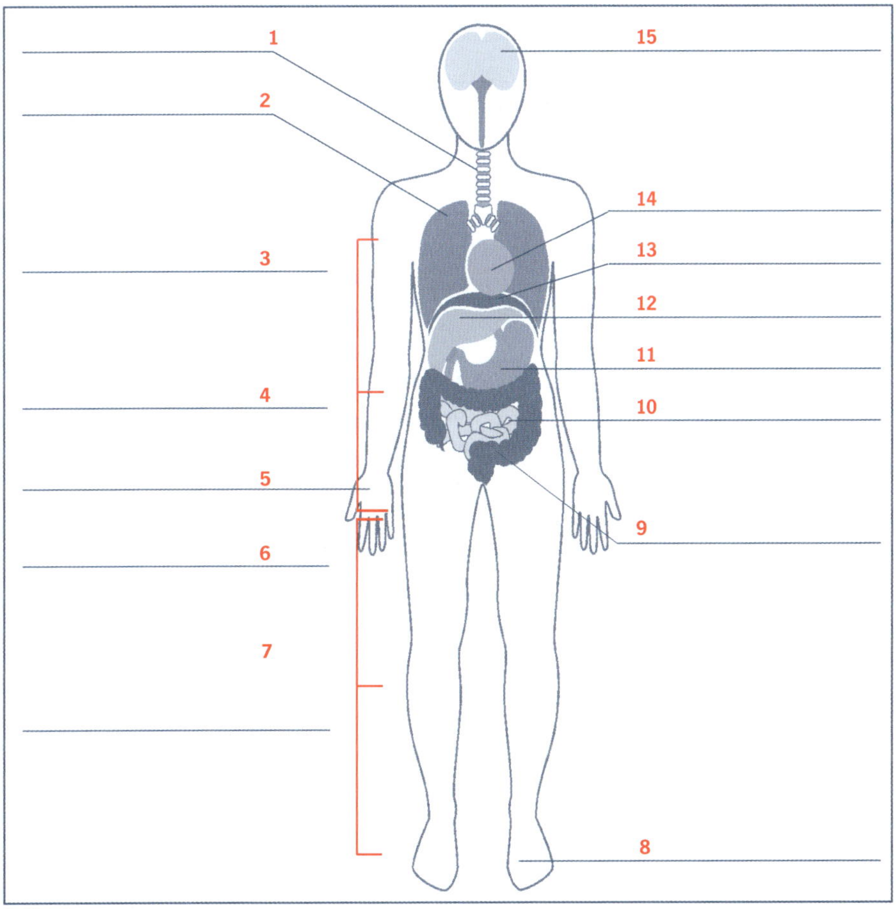

© C.K.

https://www.lienmini.fr/angsoin01

Exercice 13 : Testez-vous !

Réponse p. 32

Traduisez en anglais.

1. La pharmacie est en face de l'hôpital. ....
2. À quel étage est-ce ? ....
3. Ce matin, elle travaille dans le service des soins intensifs. ....
4. D'habitude, il travaille avec nous en chirurgie. ....
5. Je vous passe l'aide-soignante. Ne quittez pas, s'il vous plaît. ....
6. La ligne du cadre de santé est occupée. ....
7. Il y a un oreiller dans votre placard. ....

Exercice 14 : Patient education

How to maintain daily hygiene

Réponse p. 32

Cochez la (les) bonne(s) affirmation(s).

	True	False
1. You should* wash your hands after you have use the toilet.		
2. You should wash your genitals and anal area every day.		
3. You should wash your face daily*.		
4. You should have a bath or a shower at least* once a week.		
5. You should brush your teeth twice a day and have regular dental checks*.		

To help you

- **should :** vous devriez, il faudrait que…
- **daily:** tous les jours, quotidiennement
- **at least:** au moins
- **check:** contrôle

https://www.lienmini.fr/angsoinq2a

Vocabulary quiz: Units, wards and departments

Réponse p. 32

Complétez chaque définition avec le terme correct.

1. In the .... disease, injury or weakness* in the joints or muscles are treated by exercises.
a) surgical ward **b)** cardiac care unit **c)** maternity ward **d)** occupational therapy unit

2. The .... is where surgical specialists diagnose, evaluate diseases of the ear, nose and throat regions.
a) A&E* **b)** recovery room **c)** operating theatre **d)** ENT department

3. The .... is a room in a hospital used for medical operations.
a) endoscopy unit **b)** operating theatre **c)** physiotherapy unit **d)** maternity ward

4. A .... is where women go to give birth to their babies.
a) intensive care unit **b)** vascular care unit
c) operating theatre **d)** paediatric unit

5. .... is the department where people who need urgent treatment are taken.
a) A&E **b)** recovery room **c)** endoscopy unit **d)** cardiac care unit

https://www.lienmini.fr/angsoinq2b

Anatomy quiz: The body

Réponse p. 32

Complétez chaque affirmation avec le terme correct.

1. The .... is the organ inside the head that controls movement, thought*, memory and feeling.
a) stomach **b)** leg **c)** brain **d)** small intestine

2. The .... is the organ in the chest* that sends blood around the body.
a) hand **b)** foot **c)** diaphragm **d)** heart

3. The .... is the organ that cleans the blood and produces bile.
a) liver **b)** thigh **c)** trachea **d)** lung

4. The .... is either the two organs in the chest that you use for breathing.
a) forearm **b)** lung
c) upper arm **d)** hand

5. The .... is the tube in the throat that carries air to the lungs.
a) feet **b)** windpipe
c) leg **d)** thigh

To help you

- **weakness:** fragilité
- **A&E (accident and emergency):** urgences
- **thought:** pensée
- **chest:** poitrine

Medical Vocabulary: unit 2

- **chemist's shop/drugstore/pharmacy:** pharmacie
- **surgeon:** chirurgien
- **geriatric ward:** service de gériatrie
- **intensive care unit:** unité de soins intensifs
- **short-stay:** séjour de courte durée
- **out-patient:** malade en consultation externe/ambulatoire
- **operating-theatre:** bloc opératoire
- **ENT:** ORL (oto-rhino-laryngologue)

Let's discuss!

Case study

In the Accident and Emergency department, a doctor asks a nurse to insert a vesical catheter into a patient with an adenoma of the prostate. The nurse is reticent about doing it because of legal risks, but the doctor insists.

In your opinion, what could be done to avoid a situation such as this?

Exercice 2

1. Go straight on.
2. Turn left.
3. At the end of the corridor.
4. Near/Next to.
5. On your right.
6. Opposite.
7. On the third floor.

Exercice 3

1. Are you visiting him on the geriatric ward this week?
2. Is the surgeon operating next Friday?
3. Are you coming to this hospital next month?
4. Is she working in this unit at the moment?
5. What is this patient having for lunch today?

Exercice 4

1. are you doing
2. am packing
3. am leaving
4. don't understand
5. are you leaving
6. don't want
7. are you going
8. is waiting
9. are going

Exercice 5

1. to bring somebody **along** = **C.** amener quelqu'un avec soi
2. to come **up to** = **B.** venir/monter à
3. to go **down** = **A.** descendre
4. to run **into** = **E.** rentrer dans (collision)
5. to get **out of** bed = **G.** se lever
6. to run **away** = **D.** partir en courant
7. to come **from** = **F.** venir de
8. to go **to** = **J.** aller à
9. to push **through** = **K.** se frayer, s'ouvrir un chemin
10. to run **across** = **I.** traverser en courant
11. to take **along** = **H.** emmener (une personne)
12. to walk **around** = **M.** faire le tour
13. to turn **left/right** = **L.** tourner à gauche/à droite

Exercice 6

1. There is a disabled person **among** us. Please be kind and help her.
2. The pharmacy is **opposite** the operating room.
3. The bus stop is **in front of** the entrance of the hospital.
4. Mrs Parker is getting **into** the taxi.
5. I was working **on** the 8th floor of the hospital.
6. The walkway is **behind** this building.
7. Have you looked **under** the bed?
8. He sat **next to/near** me.
9. I'm looking **through** the window.
10. Please lie down **on** the bed.
11. Now I can walk **along** the corridor.
12. You can sit **between** these two patients.

Exercice 7

1. The water came **above** their knees.
2. There is a clinic **opposite** our house.
3. There were ambulances **along** the road.
4. I can't see him, he is standing **behind** the wall.
5. The room **below** is free.
6. Please, come and sit down **next/near to** me.

Corrigés

Exercice 8

1. How can I help you?
2. Who is calling, please?
3. The line's busy.
4. ... to call me back as soon as possible.
5. I'll pass on your message.

Exercice 9

1. The patient is in the antenatal ward.
2. The patient is in E.N.T.
3. The patient is in the radiography department.

Exercice 10

1. Take the lift to the 1st floor, go down the corridor, it's the 2nd door on your left.
2. Take the lift to the 3rd floor, turn right, it's the 1st door on your left.
3. Take the lift to the 3rd floor, turn right, it's the 2nd door on your left.

Exercice 11

1. She is not (isn't) in charge of the cardiac care unit.
2. He does not (doesn't) work in the psychiatric wing.
3. They never ring the bell.
4. The nursing auxiliary is not (isn't) on duty tonight.
5. Don't run in the corridor.

Exercice 12

1. windpipe/trachea
2. lung
3. upper arm
4. forearm
5. hand
6. thigh
7. leg
8. foot/feet
9. colon
10. small intestine
11. stomach
12. liver
13. diaphragm
14. heart
15. brain

Exercice 13 : Testez-vous !

1. The chemist/pharmacy is opposite the hospital.
2. Which floor is it on?
3. This morning she is working in the intensive care unit.
4. He usually works with us on the surgical ward.
5. I'll put you through to the nursing auxiliary/healthcare assistant (GB)/nurse's aid (US). Hold on, please.
6. The senior nurse's line is busy.
7. There is a pillow in the cupboard.

Exercice 14

1. True
2. True
3. True
4. False
5. True

Vocabulary quiz: Units, wards and departments

1. occupational therapy unit
2. ENT department
3. operating theatre
4. paediatric unit
5. A&E

Anatomy quiz: The body

1. brain
2. heart
3. liver
4. lung
5. windpipe

UNIT 3

UNIT 3

Dressing a wound

Toutes les pistes audio de l'unité à télécharger ici
https://www.lienmini.fr/angsoinu3

Piste 11

Dialogue between Mr Brown and the nurse

Traduction pp. 206-207

Listen to the dialogue. Mr Brown had an operation two days ago to reduce his fracture; he is in the orthopaedic ward. The surgeon has cut a window in the plaster to dress his wound*. Mr Brown's wound is purulent. His dressings are changed twice a day. Sally, a student nurse, is talking to Mr Brown's nurse. She is going to change his dressing.

Nurse Sally, let's go through the procedure together and then you can change Mr Brown's dressing. So, what do you do first?

Student Nurse First, I introduce myself to the patient and then I put on some gloves to prevent any germs getting into the wound.

Nurse Why?

Student Nurse Because this could cause infection. Then I clean the wound with some anti-septic and apply a sterile compress.

Nurse And what is the drain for?

Student Nurse It's to remove the pus.

Nurse OK, good. And what happens in the case of infection?

Student Nurse Well, we take samples* with a sterile cotton swab* and send them to the lab.

Nurse That's right. When will you remove the drain?

Student Nurse I'll remove it little by little, when the wound is no longer purulent. If this is the case, then I'll ask the surgeon to have a look first.

Nurse And what about Mr Brown's clips*? Sorry, his stitches*?

Student Nurse I'll remove the stitches in two or three days.

Nurse What do you use to remove them?

Student Nurse It depends, a stitch cutter, scissors or we can use a scalpel or a blade*.

Nurse Good. So Sally, are you ready to change Mr Brown's dressing?

Student Nurse Sure, OK.

Nurse I'll be with you in case you need my help.

Later with Mr Brown.

Nurse Is your wife coming today, Mr Brown?

Mr Brown Yes, she is coming this afternoon. She worries a lot you know. Could you cheer her up a little*? She is so anxious.

Nurse Of course, I'll talk to her when she arrives.

To help you

- **wound:** plaie
- **to do a dressing/to dress a wound:** faire un pansement
- **sample:** prélèvement
- **cotton-swab:** coton-tige pour prélèvement
- **clips:** agrafes
- **stitches:** points de suture
- **blade:** lame
- **to cheer somebody up:** réconforter quelqu'un

Questions sur le dialogue

1. Describe Mr Brown's wound. ....
2. Why is the nurse wearing gloves? ....
3. What does the nurse need to do the dressings? ....
4. What will she do if there is an infection? ....
5. What equipment does the nurse need to remove the stitches? ....
6. Why does Mr Brown want the nurse to meet his wife? ....

3 UNIT

GRAMMAR

Futur

1. Will

• Emploi

– Pour parler d'actions dont on est sûr qu'elles se produiront : I will remove your clips tomorrow.
– Pour exprimer une prévision ou une attente au sujet du futur : A lot of people will live up to the age of 100 in 2025.
– Pour exprimer une décision prise de façon soudaine : You look tired, I will get you a cup of tea.
– Pour faire une promesse ou une invitation : Don't worry, I will call you tonight.
– Pas de futur après, when, as soon as, while mais un présent : She says she will call me when she arrives.

• Construction

Forme affirmative	Forme négative	Forme interrogative
Sujet + will (she'll) + infinitif sans "to"	Sujet + will not (won't) + infinitif sans "to"	(Mot interrogatif +) will + sujet + infinitif sans "to"
She will (she'll) come tomorrow.	It will not (won't) be possible to see the doctor today.	– Will you come with me?

2. Be going to

• Emploi

Pour exprimer une intention, une décision déjà prise, ou prédire quelque chose à partir d'indices visibles, on utilise be going to.

• Construction

Forme affirmative	Forme négative	Forme interrogative
Sujet + be going to + infinitif sans "to"	Sujet + be not going to + infinitif sans "to"	Be + sujet + going to + infinitif sans "to"
I am going to give you an injection.	She is not going to work this afternoon.	Is she going to sleep here tonight?

3. To be about to

Le futur imminent peut également s'exprimer avec be about to (être sur le point de) :
– I am about to leave.
– Are you about to leave?

La forme négative "I'm not about to" a une connotation péjorative. Elle signifie « Je n'ai pas envie de ».

Exercice 1

Réponse p. 44

Complétez avec *will*, *going to* ou *about to*.

1. I .... (*be back*) tomorrow at seven.
2. She .... (*see*) the new doctor tonight.
3. Hurry up! The meeting .... (*start*).
4. Listen! The phone is ringing. I .... (*answer*) it.

Travaillez à deux

A colleague is leaving tomorrow on holiday. You're asking him/her about his/her future plans.
A. Where are you going on holiday this year? **B.** I haven't decided yet/I haven't made up my mind. I might go to Scotland or Finland.

Complétez les questions de A à l'aide des éléments de réponses de B, puis rédigez les réponses de B.

1. **A.** How .... travel?
   B. By plane./By boat.
2. **A.** Where .... stay?
   B. At friend's./In a bed and breakfast.
3. **A.** How long .... stay?
   B. For a fortnight./For a week.
4. **A.** Who .... go with?
   B. My husband./My wife./Alone.

Exercice 2

Réponse p. 44

Complétez la légende à l'aide des mots suivants :

- dermis
- cornified layer
- sweat gland
- arteriole
- sebaceous gland
- venule
- pore
- adipose tissue
- arrector pili muscle
- hair follicle
- hair
- epidermis

The skin

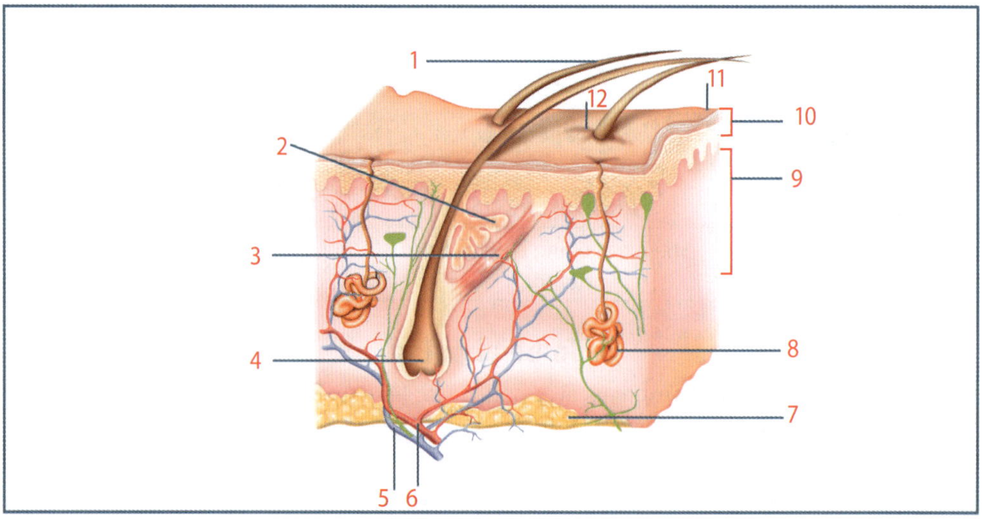

https://www.lienmini.fr/angsoin04

Exercice 3 : Requests and offers

Réponse p. 44

Suivez les instructions suivantes (A et B).

A. is a nurse or a nursing auxiliary.
B. is the patient. He has several requests.

Ex.:
Nurse: *Can I help you?*
Patient: *Certainly. It's hot. Could you open the window, please?*
Nurse: *Sorry, you want me to open the window, do you?*
Patient: *Yes, please.*

1. It's hot in his room. (*Il demande à l'infirmière d'ouvrir la fenêtre.*)

....

2. He can't sleep. (*Il demande un somnifère.*)

....

3. The light is hurting his eyes. (*Il demande de baisser le rideau.*)

....

4. His leg is painful. (*Il demande un antalgique.*)

....

5. He thinks he has a temperature. (*Il demande un thermomètre.*)

....

6. He wants to urinate. (*Il demande l'urinal.*)

....

GRAMMAR

Articles

1. L'article indéfini : a/an

• Emploi

A + consonne	An + voyelle
a car, a nurse, a patient. Exceptions : an hour, an honest person, an honour.	an apple. Exceptions : a uniform, a European.

• Remarques

On utilise l'article a/an :
– devant les professions : I am a surgeon;
– après what et such suivis d'un nom au singulier : What a great surgeon!
– dans certaines expressions : I have a headache and a sore throat.

2. L'article défini : the

• Emploi

On l'utilise pour parler de quelque chose de spécifique : I like the people in this country.
On le supprime pour parler de généralités : I like people.

• Remarques

Quelques cas particuliers :
- on the radio, listen to the radio, watch television;
- the poor, the rich, the dead, the disabled, etc.

Exercice 4

Réponse p. 44

Complétez avec *the* si nécessaire ou laissez un blanc.

1. ....life has always been difficult for .... poor.
2. In Africa .... life of AIDS patients is getting more and more difficult.
3. .... lung cancer is often linked to tobacco smoking.
4. .... high cholesterol runs in families*.
5. What are .... most common childhood diseases? .... measles, ... German measles, ... mumps and .... chickenpox.
6. .... flu is a contagious disease.

To help you

- **to run in families:** se transmettre de génération en génération

Exercice 5

Réponse p. 44

Complétez avec *a* ou *an*.

1. My son has got .... bad cold.
2. His uncle is such .... great surgeon.
3. What .... excellent midwife her aunt is!
4. .... thermometer is .... instrument for measuring temperature.
5. What .... pity!

Piste 12

Exercice 6 : Urinating

Traduction p. 207
Réponse p. 44

Écoutez le dialogue.
Puis complétez la conversation entre l'infirmier et la patiente. Utilisez les phrases suivantes :

- on the bedpan
- Use the bell to call me
- Your urine seems to be cloudy
- ... to have a wee
- a drainage bag
- it burns a little
- ... when passing urine?
- I'll insert the tube gently ...

Nurse Do you need anything?

Patient (ill at ease) I'd like to pass, er.... to pass water...

Nurse I'm sorry but I don't understand.

Patient Er... I'd like **(1)** ....

Nurse Oh, sorry, you mean you need to go to the toilet.

Patient Yes. Exactly.

Nurse I'll put you **(2)** ....
Here is some toilet paper. **(3)** ....
when you have finished.

Patient Thank you.

Nurse You're welcome.

A few minutes later.

Nurse **(4)** .... , so I'll send a specimen* to the lab later on. Do you have any problems **(5)** ....

Patient Not really, but **(6)** ....

The following day.

Nurse The doctor wants you to have a catheter. Don't worry. **(7)** .... into your bladder, then I'll attach **(8)** .... to collect the urine.

To help you

- **specimen:** échantillon pour les urines

Piste 13

Exercice 7

Réponse p. 45

Écoutez, puis répétez.
Complétez la légende à l'aide des mots suivants :

- pad/nappy
- specimen bottle
- catheter
- bladder
- kidney
- urinal
- drainage bag

Urinating

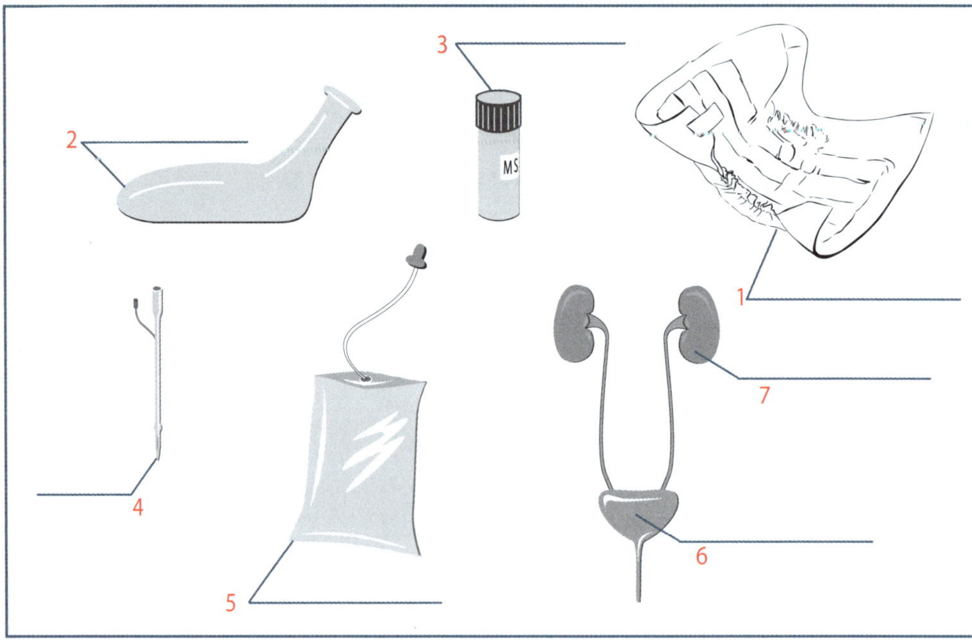

https://www.lienmini.fr/angsoin05

Piste 14

Travaillez à deux

Réponse p. 45

Écoutez, puis répétez.
Lisez attentivement les mots suivants, puis utilisez-les pour répondre aux questions de votre partenaire :

- throat
- elbow
- trunk
- bladder
- skin
- shoulder

A asks B:

1. What is the name of the organ which contains urine? ....
2. What is the name of the joint between the upper arm and the forearm? ....
3. What is the name of the natural covering of the body? ....

B asks A:

4. Where are the tonsils situated? ....
5. Where are the ribs located? ....
6. Where is the clavicle situated? ....

Exercice 8

Réponse p. 45

Complétez la légende à l'aide des mots suivants :

- forceps/tweezers
- scissors
- antiseptic
- swab/compress
- stitch cutter
- scalpel

Equipment for dressing a wound

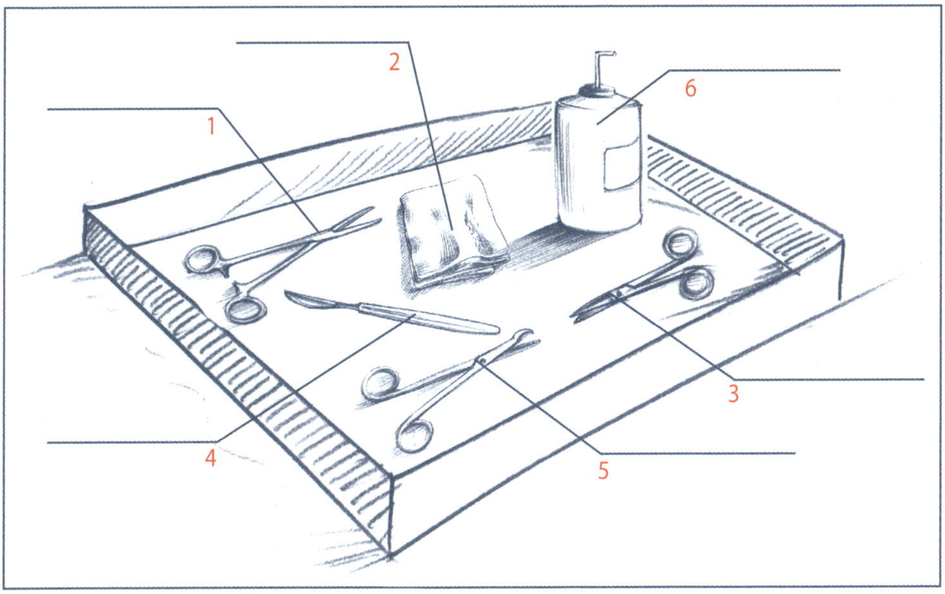

© C.K.

https://www.lienmini.fr/angsoin06

Exercice 9 : Testez-vous !

Réponse p. 45

Traduisez en anglais.

1. Quand enlèverez-vous mes points ? ....

2. J'enlèverai le drain lorsque le docteur me le dira. ....

3. Dépêchez-vous ! Ils sont sur le point d'arriver. ....

4. Pourriez-vous me donner le bassin, s'il vous plaît. J'ai besoin d'uriner. ....

5. Appelez-moi quand vous aurez fini. ....

6. Vos urines sont troubles. Je vais envoyer un échantillon aux laboratoires. ....

7. Je vais poser une sonde urinaire. ....

Exercice 10 : Care delivery

Réponse p. 45

Therapeutic relationships

Cochez la (les) bonne(s) affirmation(s).

	True	False
1. Nurses do not need to maximize the time they spend on patient education to obtain the best outcomes* for their patients.		
2. For patient teaching to be effective*, nurses must know their patients and individualize patient education.		
3. Create surroundings* that support teaching and engage the learner and an environment that makes the patient comfortable.		
4. Be sure not to use the same kind of equipment the patient will be using at home.		
5. The nurse can have the patient verbalize what has been learned. The goal of effective teaching is to say: "Tell and show me what you understand."		

To help you

- **outcome :** résultat
- **effective :** efficace
- **surrounding :** environnement

https://www.lienmini.fr/angsoinq3a

Vocabulary quiz: Medical equipment* and tools*

Réponse p. 45

Complétez chaque définition avec le terme correct.

1. The .... is the liquid used to sterelize the skin.
a) essential oil **b)** gauze **c)** antiseptic **d)** ether

2. A .... is a piece of material placed over a wound to protect it.
a) monitor **b)** tube **c)** dressing **d)** bandage

3. A .... is a cloth covering that is placed over a wound to prevent infection and bleeding.
a) needle **b)** bandage **c)** dressing **d)** thermometer

4. The .... is the tool that measures the force of blood flow*.
a) IV bag **b)** monitor **c)** scales **d)** blood pressure monitor

5. The .... is used for taking blood or administering medicine.
a) glass cylinder **b)** needle **c)** screen **d)** thermometer

https://www.lienmini.fr/angsoinq3b

Verbs quiz: Dressing a wound

Réponse p. 45

Complétez chaque affirmation avec le verbe correct.

1. Don't forget to .... some gloves before dressing a wound.
a) remove **b)** put on **c)** use **d)** put off

2. To .... the stitches you use a stitch cutter, a blade or a scalpel.
a) put **b)** do **c)** make **d)** remove

3. You must .... the wound with some antiseptic.
a) clear **b)** clean **c)** wash **d)** change

4. Sorry, I'm not ready to .... his dressing right now.
a) cut **b)** change **c)** take **d)** send

5. They have to .... the samples to the lab before 10:30.
a) put **b)** clean **c)** send **d)** use

To help you

- **equipment:** matériel
- **tool:** instrument, outil
- **blood flow:** circulation sanguine

Medical Vocabulary: unit 3

- **wound:** plaie
- **stitches:** points de suture
- **to do a dressing:** faire un pansement
- **gloves:** gants
- **forearm:** avant-bras
- **bedpan:** bassin
- **bladder:** vessie
- **forceps/tweezers:** pinces/forceps
- **rib:** côte
- **elbow:** coude
- **tonsils:** amygdales

Let's discuss!

Patient education

How could you educate patients in a more effective manner? Give two examples.

Corrigés

Exercice 1

1. I **will** be back tomorrow at seven.
2. She **is going to** see the new doctor tonight.
3. Hurry up! The meeting **is about to** start.
4. Listen! The phone is ringing. I **will** answer it.

Exercice 2

1. hair
2. sebaceous gland
3. arrector pilli muscle
4. hair follicle
5. venule
6. arteriole
7. adipose tissue
8. sweat gland
9. dermis
10. epidermis
11. cornified layer
12. pore

Exercice 3

1. B. It's hot. Could you open the window, please?
   A. Sorry, you want me to open the window, do you?
2. B. Could you give me a sleeping pill, please?
   A. Sorry, you want me to give you a sleeping pill, do you?
3. B. Could you lower the blind, please?
   A. Sorry, you want me to lower the blind, do you?
4. B. Could you give me a painkiller, please?
   A. Sorry, you want me to give you a painkiller, do you?
5. B. Could you give me a thermometer, please?
   A. Sorry, you want me to give you a thermometer, do you?
6. B. Could you give me the urinal, please?
   A. Sorry, you want me to give you the urinal, do you?

Exercice 4

1. **Life** has always been difficult for **the** poor.
2. In Africa **the** life of AIDS patients is getting more and more difficult.
3. **Lung cancer** is often linked to tobacco smoking.
4. **High cholesterol** runs in families.
5. What are **the** most common childhood diseases? **Measles**, **German measles**, **mumps** and **chickenpox**.
6. **The** flu is a contagious disease.

Exercice 5

1. My son has got **a** bad cold.
2. His uncle is such **a** great surgeon.
3. What **an** excellent midwife her aunt is!
4. **A** thermometer is **an** instrument for measuring temperature.
5. What **a** pity!

Exercice 6

1. to have a wee.
2. on the bedpan.
3. Use the bell to call me
4. Your urine seems to be cloudy
5. when passing urine?
6. it burns a little.
7. I'll insert the tube gently
8. a drainage bag

Corrigés

Exercice 7

1. pad/nappy
2. urinal
3. specimen bottle
4. catheter
5. drainage bag
6. bladder
7. kidney

Travaillez à deux

1. bladder
2. elbow
3. skin
4. throat
5. trunk
6. shoulder

Exercice 8

1. forceps/tweezers
2. swab/compress
3. scissors
4. scalpel
5. stitch cutter
6. antiseptic

Exercice 9 : Testez-vous !

1. When will you remove my stitches?
2. I'll remove the drain when the doctor tells me.
3. Hurry up! They are about to come/arrive.
4. Could you give me the bedpan, please? I need to have a wee/ to urinate/to pass water.
5. Call me when you have finished.
6. Your urine is cloudy. I'm going to send a specimen to the lab.
7. I'm going to insert a urinary tube/catheter.

Exercice 10

1. False
2. True
3. True
4. False
5. True

Vocabulary quiz: Medical equipment and tools

1. antiseptic
2. dressing
3. bandage
4. blood pressure monitor
5. needle

Verbs quiz: Dressing a wound

1. put on
2. remove
3. clean
4. change
5. send

UNIT 4

UNIT 4

Obtaining information about antecedents

Toutes les pistes audio de l'unité à télécharger ici
https://www.lienmini.fr/angsoinu4

Piste 15

Dialogue between Mrs Brown and Dr Lavau

Traduction p. 208

Listen to the dialogue. Mr Brown had heart complications yesterday. Doctor Lavau is asking Mrs Brown some general questions about her husband's personal history. He wants to know if there are any particular antecedents in his family.

Dr Lavau Do you know if there is a problem of high blood pressure in his family?

Mrs Brown No, I don't think so.

Dr Lavau Are there any cases of heart attacks or strokes*?

Mrs Brown He once told me his grandfather on his mother's side died of a sudden heart attack. As for his parents, his father died three years ago.

Dr Lavau What did he die of?

Mrs Brown He died of lung cancer*.

Dr Lavau Is your husband a heavy smoker*?

Mrs Brown Yes, he is. He smokes 25 cigarettes a day, at least...

Dr Lavau Yesterday, I saw on his medical record* he has angina. Does he do any sport or regular exercise?

Mrs Brown He does a lot of gardening, but that's all.

Dr Lavau Did he have any chest* pain before yesterday?

Mrs Brown Yes, but he thought it was nothing serious although I told him it could be. A few months ago, I noticed he was short of breath*.

Dr Lavau Thank you very much, Mrs Brown.

To help you

- **stroke:** attaque d'apoplexie
- **lung cancer:** cancer du poumon
- **heavy smoker:** gros fumeur
- **medical record:** dossier médical
- **chest:** poitrine
- **to be short of breath:** s'essouffler/manquer d'air

Questions sur le dialogue

1. What happened to Mr Brown yesterday? ....

....

....

2. Why does Doctor Lavau want to meet his wife? ....

....

....

3. What did Mr Brown's grandfather die of? ....

....

4. In your opinion, what is Mr Brown's attitude about his health? ....

....

....

5. What are Mr Brown's risk factors? ....

....

....

GRAMMAR

Past simple (prétérit)

• Emploi

On utilise le past simple (prétérit) pour parler du passé quand les actions, les faits, sont terminés.
Il correspond généralement au passé composé français.
Il s'emploie souvent avec des marqueurs de temps tels que : yesterday, last week, ago, in 2002.

• Construction des phrases

Forme affirmative	Forme négative	Forme interrogative
Sujet + verbe régulier + -ed Sujet + verbe irrégulier (liste p. 185)	Sujet + did not (didn't) + verbe	Did + sujet + verbe
She lived near the hospital. I told him the truth.	She didn't take her temperature yesterday.	Did you work on this ward last year? – Yes, I did. – No, I didn't.

• Remarques

- On ajoute un -d aux verbes qui se terminent en -e (to arrive = arrived) ou -ed aux verbes qui se terminent par une consonne (to start = started).
- Pour les verbes se terminant par une consonne + y, le y se change en i (to try = tried). Le y ne change pas lorsqu'il est précédé d'une voyelle (to play = played).
- Prononciation :
  . après les sons /t/ et /d,/ -ed se prononce [id] ;
  . après les sons /f/, /k/, /p/, /s/ et /S/ (= ch), le -ed se prononce [t]. Il se prononce [d] dans les autres cas, notamment après les voyelles.

Exercice 1

Réponse p. 60

Posez les questions afin d'obtenir les réponses écrites en bleu.

1. She had an X-ray taken **last week**.
2. A meeting took place last night **to discuss Mrs White's case**.
3. I did not phone her **because her results weren't back from the lab yet**.
4. He did not take his medication **because he is allergic to antibiotics**.
5. He didn't come **because he cancelled his appointment yesterday**.

Travaillez à deux

Discutez des trois situations suivantes. Vous pouvez vous aider des phrases interrogatives ci-après. A est une infirmière qui pose des questions à sa collègue B. Changez de rôle à chaque situation.

1. A patient who arrived last week.
2. An accident which happened yesterday.
3. A young girl who had an operation this morning.

Questions :

1. When did he arrive exactly?
   Who was he with?
   Why did he come to the hospital?
2. Where was it?
   When did it happen?
   What happened next?
3. Were there any complications during the operation?
   Was her mother with her? (No) Why not?
   Did you check these vital signs (blood pressure, pulse, temperature and respiration rate)?

Exercice 2 : Declining an offer

Réponse p. 60

Improvisez un dialogue en utilisant les amorces suivantes.

Ex.: A drink.

A. Would you like a drink? **B.** No thanks, I'm not thirsty.

1. Some biscuits.
2. To talk.
3. To watch television.
4. An extra pillow.
5. To walk to the TV room.

GRAMMAR

Adverbes et adverbes de fréquence

• Adverbes

– Les adverbes se forment à partir des adjectifs auxquels on ajoute -ly.

. Ex.: The new nurse works quickly.

. slow + ly - slowly / intelligent + -ly - intelligently.

– Pour les adjectifs se terminant par -y, on change le -y en -i et on ajoute -ly : happy - happily.

– Pour les adjectifs se terminant par -le, on supprime le -e et on le remplace par -y : simple - simply.

– Pour les adjectifs se terminant par -ll, on ajoute -y : full - fully

Quelques exceptions : good – well / fast – fast / hard – hard.

Les adverbes se placent après le verbe : She speaks (English) well.

• Adverbes de fréquence

Every day: tous les jours
Every other day: tous les deux jours
At bedtime: à l'heure du coucher
From time to time: de temps en temps
Before/after meals: avant/après les repas
At mealtimes: à l'heure des repas
Last: en dernier/pour la dernière fois
3 or 4 times daily: 3 à 4 fois par jour.

Les adverbes de fréquence se placent :

– Presque toujours entre le sujet et le verbe : This doctor often sees patients at home.

– Après l'auxiliaire être : She was always late.

– Après l'auxiliaire avoir (quand il est conjugué) : He has never left this ward.

Exercice 3

Réponse p. 60

Placez au bon endroit les adverbes entre parenthèses dans les phrases suivantes.

1. She is upset when she doesn't have visitors (*often*). She ....

....

2. He takes his medication (*rarely*). He ....

....

3. She complains about the food (*sometimes*). She ....

....

4. He is in a bad mood (*never*). He ....

....

5. She speaks politely to the nurses (*usually*). She ....

....

Travaillez à deux

Posez ces questions à votre partenaire, inscrivez ses réponses ; puis inversez les rôles.

1. How often did you see your GP last year? ....
....
2. Why did you see your GP last year? ....
....
3. When did you last take your temperature? ....
....
4. What did you take the last time you had a headache? ....
....
5. When did you last have an X-ray? ....
....

GRAMMAR

L'impératif

• Emploi

L'impératif est un mode verbal qui sert à exprimer le commandement, l'exhortation, le conseil, la prière et la défense.

• Construction

Forme affirmative	verbe	Call the nurse, please.
Forme négative	Do + not (don't) + verbe	Do not (don't) touch her leg.

• Remarque

Pour donner plus de force à la phrase, on peut utiliser l'expression make sure + sujet + verbe à la forme impérative.
– Make sure you close the door.

Piste 16

Exercice 4

Réponse p. 60

Écoutez les injonctions données par un médecin en vue d'un examen, puis faites-les correspondre à leurs équivalents français ci-dessous.

Détendez-vous : ....
Allongez-vous : ....
Ouvrez la bouche : ....
Ouvrez les yeux : ....
Suivez mon doigt : ....
Avalez : ....
Respirez profondément : ....

Asseyez-vous : ....
Levez-vous : ....
Toussez : ....
Fermez les yeux : ....
Poussez : ....
Ne respirez plus : ....

Exercice 5 : Pain

Piste 17

Traduction p. 208
Réponse p. 60

Écoutez le dialogue et complétez la conversation entre l'infirmière et le patient. Utilisez les phrases suivantes :

- a slight headache...
- where it hurts.
- What kind of pain is it?
- a sharp pain or a dull pain?
- I can give you a painkiller ...
- it won't hurt so much tomorrow.

Nurse How are you today?

Patient I don't feel very well. My knee hurts.

Nurse (1) ....

Patient It's hard to tell.

Nurse Is it (2) ....

Patient I can't explain exactly. It's a constant pain.

Nurse Could you show me (3) ....

Patient Right here.

Nurse If the pain continues, I'll ask the doctor if (4) .... to relieve the pain.

Patient I've got (5) .... too. I feel so tired today.

Nurse It's quite normal, you know. You had an operation yesterday. Don't worry, (6) ....

Exercice 6 : Pain

Piste 18

Réponse p. 60

Écoutez la piste 18 qui vous donnera des informations sur l'expression de la douleur (vous pouvez suivre en lisant le texte ci-dessous).

How to describe pain.

His leg is painful (he has got a pain in his leg). His knee hurts. He has got a sore throat...

The degree of pain varies a lot from one person to another. The patient may use different adjectives to describe the type of pain he or she feels. This can be helpful to diagnose an illness. Here is a list of useful adjectives.

Traduisez les termes suivants en français :

constant pain: ....
intermittent pain: ....
dull pain: ....
general pain: ....
sharp pain: ....
severe pain: ....
recurrent pain: ....
burning pain: ....
localized pain: ....
slight pain: ....

Piste 19

Exercice 7

Réponse p. 60

Écoutez, puis répétez.
Complétez la légende avec les mots suivants.

- shoulder
- knee
- ankle
- wrist
- elbow
- hip
- foot/feet
- hand
- neck
- jaw

Articulations/joints

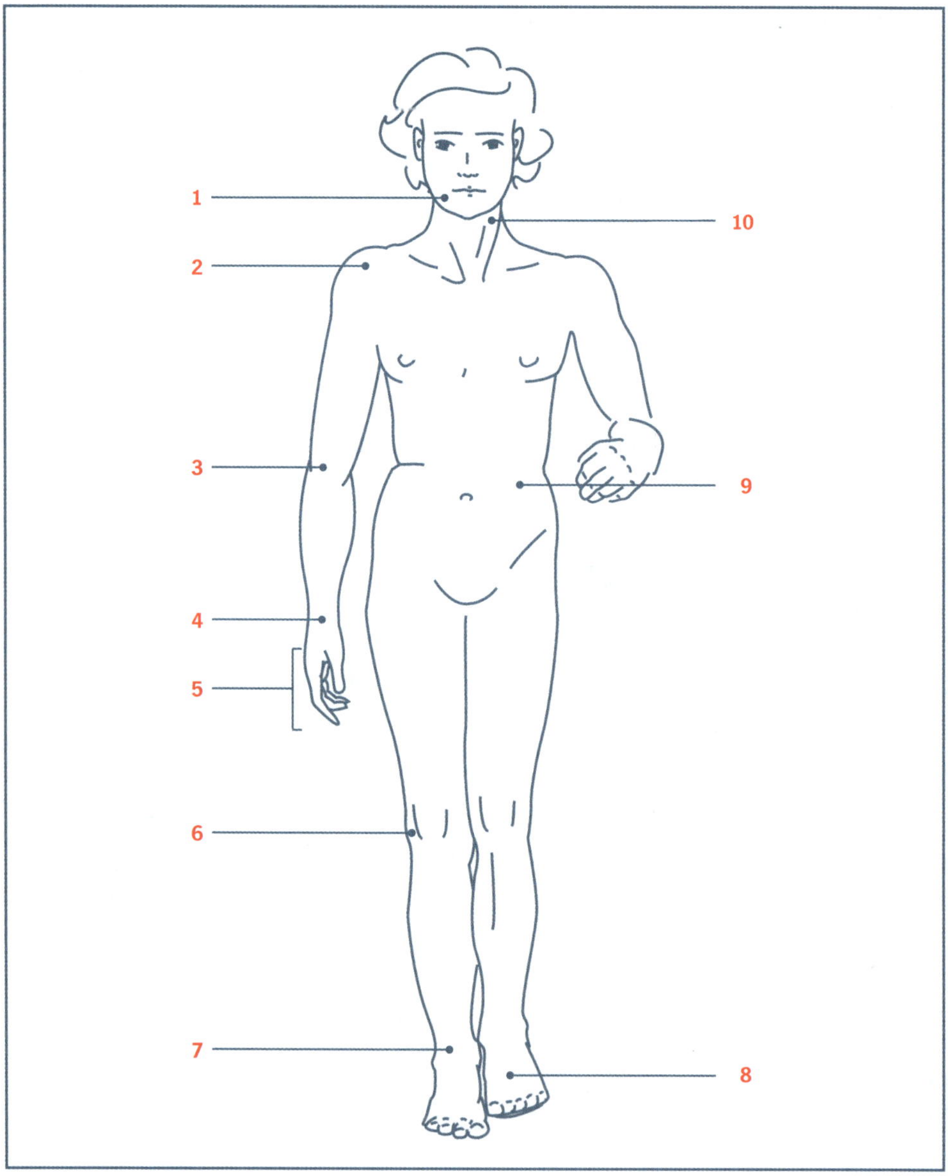

https://www.lienmini.fr/angsoin07

GRAMMAR

Exprimer la cause

• Emploi

On utilise :

- for et to pour parler de l'utilité d'un objet : A syringe is used to give somebody an injection/for giving an injection;
- so that pour parler du but d'une action : He worked a lot so that everything would be ready in time;
- to pour parler du but également mais avec une construction différente : To get better, you must take your medication;
- because pour expliquer la raison d'une action citée juste avant : He walked with crutches because he had broken his leg;
- that's why pour exprimer une conséquence : You had an operation; that's why you have to stay in hospital.

• Construction

For	For + nom For + verbe en-ing	This city is famous for its hospital. A blade is for removing stitches.
To	To + infinitif	This medicine is used to cure colds.
So that	So that + préposition	I will clean your wound so that you don't get an infection.
Because	Because + raison	I am tired because I didn't sleep well last night.
That's why	That's why + conséquence	You are dehydrated; that's why you need to drink lots of water.

Exercice 8

Réponse p. 61

Complétez les phrases ci-dessous avec les expressions suivantes :

• that's why	• for	• to
• because	• so	• so that

1. This treatment is often given .... cure this disease.
2. I had forgotten my phone yesterday, ... I couldn't call you.
3. I can't take these pills .... I have an allergy.
4. You should explain it to me, ... I will be able to help you.
5. This equipment can be very useful .... the medical staff.
6. The room was full .... they moved him to a new one.

Exercice 9

Réponse p. 61

Complétez la légende avec les mots suivants :

- probe
- splint
- scalpel
- syringe
- pin
- wheelchair

Medical equipment

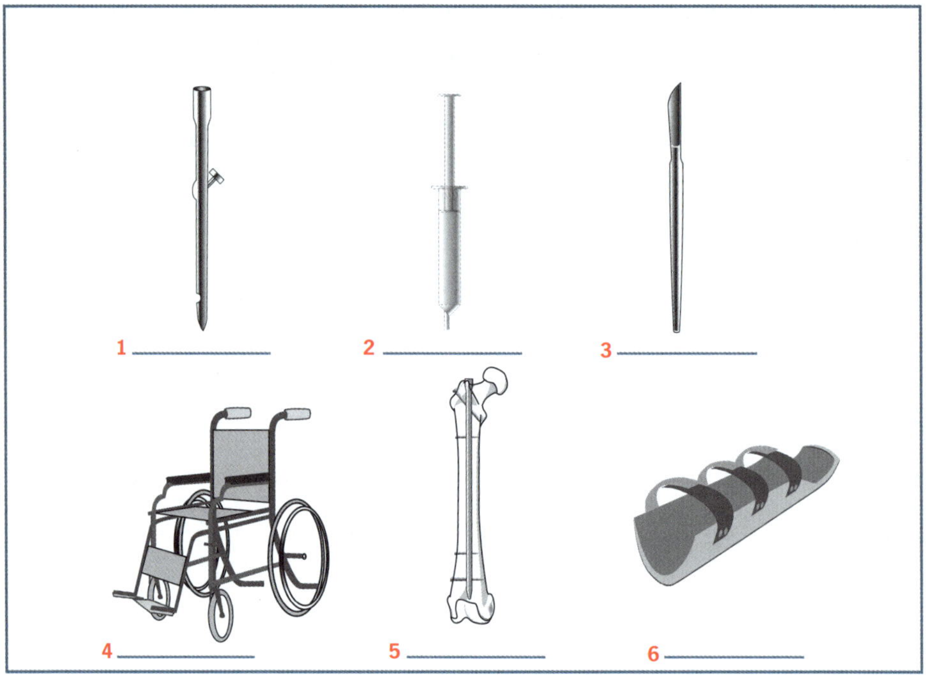

https://www.lienmini.fr/angsoin08

Exercice 10

Réponse p. 61

Faites correspondre les mots suivants à la définition qui leur convient :

- pin
- splint
- syringe
- scalpel
- probe
- wheelchair

1. A .... is an instrument with a fine needle for injections.
2. A .... is an instrument used to explore inside a wound.
3. A .... is a chair in which the disabled can move around.
4. A .... is a piece of metal to fasten together parts of a broken bone.
5. A .... is a piece of metal which is fastened to a broken leg or arm to keep it in the same position.
6. A .... is a short knife used by surgeons.

Exercice 11 : Testez-vous !

Réponse p. 61

Traduisez en anglais.

1. Elle oublie de prendre ses gélules de temps en temps. ....

2. L'année dernière, je prenais de la pénicilline deux fois par jour à l'heure des repas. ....

3. L'infirmière passera tous les deux jours pour vous faire une piqûre. ....

4. J'ai une légère douleur à la jambe lorsque je marche. ....

5. Avez-vous eu mal au dos hier ? ....

6. De quoi votre mère est-elle morte ? ....

7. Quand il était interne, il n'a jamais perdu ses dossiers médicaux. ....

Exercie 12 : Patient information

Réponse p. 61

Joint pain

Cochez la (les) bonne(s) affirmation(s).

	True	False
1. Joint pain is discomfort that arises from any joint. It is sometimes called arthralgia.		
2. Sprains are injuries to the body, often resulting* from physical activity. These injuries are common and can range from minor to severe.		
3. Some causes of joint pain require treatment for a long time and cause long-term joint problems.		
4. If you have an infection in a joint then you will not need to be seen in hospital as an emergency.		
5. If you have rheumatoid arthritis then you will need an urgent appointment with a specialist because starting treatment early will reduce the risk of long-term problems.		

To help you

- **sprain :** entorse, foulure
- **to resolve :** résoudre, soulager

https://www.lienmini.fr/angsoinq4a

Vocabulary quiz: Medical equipment and tools

Réponse p. 61

Complétez chaque définition avec le terme correct.

1. The .... contains liquids to be pumped into a patient's body.
a) syringe **b)** bottle **c)** mask **d)** IV(intraveinous) bag

2. The device that measures a person's weight* is called the ....
a) scales **b)** probe **c)** screen **d)** monitor

3. The .... is used to listen to a person's heart and lungs.
a) oxymeter **b)** stetoscope
c) catheter **d)** microscope

To help you

- **weight:** poids

4. The..measures the degree of oxygen saturation of the circulating blood.
a) scalpel **b)** test tube **c)** syringe **d)** oxymeter

5. A .... is a glass cylinder filled with blood or other liquids.
a) probe **b)** test tube **c)** forceps **d)** thermomete

https://www.lienmini.fr/angsoinq4b

Anatomy quiz: Articulations/Joints

Réponse p. 61

Complétez chaque affirmation avec le terme correct.

1. The part of the body between the top of the arm and the neck is the ....
a) leg **b)** elbow **c)** knee **d)** shoulder

2. The.. is the joint between the hand and the arm.
a) jaw **b)** shoulder **c)** wrist **d)** elbow

3. The joint connecting the foot to the leg is called the ....
a) ankle **b)** foot **c)** hip **d)** jaw

4. The .... is the joint between the forearm and the upperarm.
a) hand **b)** neck **c)** arm **d)** elbow

5. The .... is the joint at the top of the leg.
a) wrist **b)** knee **c)** hip **d)** jaw

Medical Vocabulary: unit 4

- **pain:** douleur
- **painkiller:** analgésique
- **chest:** poitrine
- **probe:** sonde
- **splint:** attelle
- **to follow a treatment:** suivre un traitement
- **wrist:** poignet
- **ankle:** cheville
- **hip:** hanche
- **neck:** cou
- **medical record:** dossier médical
- **risk factors:** facteurs de risque

Let's discuss!

Pain in children.

Special Interest Group on Pain in Childhood

The IASP's (International Association for the Study of Pain) asks for "priority on pain in infants, children and adolescents."

Children's pain must become a priority for all health care professionals.

How has the measurement of pain in children advanced in the last decade? How many standardized measures do you know? How can you help relieve pain for children in hospital?

Corrigés

Exercice 1

1. When did she have an X-ray taken?
2. What did they discuss last night?/Whose case did they discuss?
3. Why didn't you phone her?
4. Why he did not take his medication?
5. Why didn't he come?

Exercice 2

1. **A.** Would you like some biscuits?
   B. No thanks, I'm not hungry.
2. **A.** Would you like to talk?
   B. No thanks, I'm too tired.
3. **A.** Would you like to watch TV?
   B. No thanks, there is nothing interesting on.
4. **A.** Would you like an extra pillow?
   B. No thanks, one is enough.
5. **A.** Would you like to walk to the TV room?
   B. No thanks, my leg hurts.

Exercice 3

1. She is **often** upset when she doesn't have visitors.
2. He **rarely** takes his medication.
3. She **sometimes** complains about the food.
4. He is **never** in a bad mood.
5. She **usually** speaks politely to the nurses.

Exercice 4

Détendez-vous : Relax
Allongez-vous : Lie down
Ouvrez la bouche : Open your mouth
Ouvrez les yeux : Open your eyes
Suivez mon doigt : Follow my finger
Avalez : Swallow
Respirez profondément : Breathe deeply
Asseyez-vous : Sit down
Levez-vous : Get up/Stand up
Toussez : Cough
Fermez les yeux : Close/Shut your eyes
Poussez : Push
Ne respirez plus : Hold your breath

Exercice 5

1. What kind of pain is it?
2. a sharp pain or a dull pain?
3. where it hurts.
4. I can give you a painkiller…
5. a slight headache…
6. it won't hurt so much tomorrow.

Exercice 6

Constant pain: douleur constante.
Intermittent pain: douleur intermittente.
Dull pain: douleur vague ou sourde.
General pain: douleur généralisée.
Sharp pain: douleur aiguë.
Severe pain: forte douleur.
Recurrent pain: douleur périodique/qui revient.
Burning pain: douleur avec sensation de brûlure.
Localized pain: douleur localisée.
Slight pain: légère douleur.

Exercice 7

1. jaw
2. shoulder
3. elbow
4. wrist
5. hand
6. knee
7. ankle
8. one foot/two feet
9. hip
10. neck

Corrigés

Exercice 8

1. This treatment is often given **to** cure this disease.
2. I had forgotten my phone yesterday, **that's why** I couldn't call you.
3. I can't take these pills **because** I have an allergy.
4. You should explain it to me, **so that** I will be able to help you.
5. This equipment can be very useful **for** the medical staff.
6. The room was full **so** they moved him to a new one.

Exercice 9

1. probe
2. syringe
3. scalpel
4. wheelchair
5. pin
6. splint

Exercice 10

1. syringe
2. probe
3. wheelchair
4. pin
5. splint
6. scalpel

Exercice 11 : Testez-vous !

1. She forgets to take her capsules from time to time.
2. Last year, I was on penicillin twice a day at meal times.
3. The nurse will come every other day to give you an injection.
4. I've got a slight pain in my leg when I walk.
5. Did your back hurt yesterday? / Was your back painful yesterday?
6. What did your mother die of?
7. He never lost his medical records when he was an intern.

Exercice 12

1. True
2. True
3. True
4. False
5. True

Vocabulary quiz: Medical equipment and tools

1. IV (intraveinous) bag
2. scales
3. stetoscope
4. oxymeter
5. test tube

Anatomy quiz: Joints/ Articulation

1. shoulder
2. wrist
3. ankle
4. elbow
5. hip

UNIT 5

UNIT 5 Clinical examination and nursing care

Toutes les pistes audio de l'unité à télécharger ici
https://www.lienmini.fr/angsoinu5

Piste 20

Dialogue between Mr Brown and Dr Martin and between Mr Brown and the healthcare assistant*

Traduction p. 209

Listen to the dialogue. Dr Martin is examining Mr Brown who has heart complications. He's explaining what he is doing.

Doctor First, I'm going to check* your heart. Could you sit down, please?

Mr Brown Yes, certainly.

Doctor Could you take off* your pyjama top, please? Thank you. Open your mouth and breathe deeply*. I want to listen to your breathing. I'm sorry, the stethoscope is cold, isn't it?

Mr Brown Yes, it is.

Doctor Breathe in and out* with your mouth open. Slowly, please. Now, cough*. That's fine. Hold your breath. Uhum. Does it hurt when I press here?

Mr Brown A little.

Doctor All right, you can get dressed* now Mr Brown. Thank you very much.

A few minutes later, a healthcare assistant comes to give Mr Brown a bedbath.

HCA It's time to have a wash*, Mr Brown. Is the water OK for you?

Mr Brown Yes, it's all right. I would like to have a shave* today.

HCA Of course. Where is your shaving cream and your razor?

Mr Brown In my locker.

HCA Tomorrow you can have a wash in the bathroom.

Mr Brown That's great! I'll have a shower* and wash my hair.

HCA Could you lift* your arm, please? Thank you. Could you turn over. I'll just rub some ointment* on your bottom if that's OK. It's to prevent bedsores*.

Mr Brown Could you put my pyjamas in this bag, please? My wife can then take them home to wash them.

To help you

- **healthcare assistant (HCA):** aide-soignante
- **to check:** vérifier
- **to take off:** enlever (un vêtement)
- **to breathe deeply:** respirer profondément
- **to breathe in and out:** inspirer, expirer
- **to cough:** tousser
- **to get dressed:** s'habiller
- **to have a wash:** se laver
- **to have a shave:** se raser
- **to have a shower:** prendre une douche
- **to lift:** lever
- **to rub on some ointment:** appliquer de la pommade
- **to prevent bedsores:** éviter les escarres

Questions sur le dialogue

1. List the verbs Dr Martin uses as he carries out the clinical examination. ....
....
....
2. At the end of this examination, what does Dr Martin ask Mr Brown to do? ....
....
....
3. List the verbs the HCA uses as she washes Mr Brown. ....
....
....
4. Why does she use ointment? ....
....
....

GRAMMAR

Present perfect

• Emploi

– Pour parler d'actions passées qui ont des conséquences sur le présent :
. The patient has seen his family today; that's why he is so tired.

– Pour parler d'actions qui ont commencé dans le passé mais qui se poursuivent dans le présent :
. He has worked in the same hospital for ten years.

– Avec les expressions de temps suivantes : ever, never, already, recently, not … yet, just, so far, this week, this month, since, when, etc. :
. I have never worked in this unit.

• Construction

Forme affirmative	Forme négative	Forme interrogative
Sujet + have/has + participe passé (verbe + -ed pour les verbes réguliers, 3e colonne du tableau p. 186 pour les verbes irréguliers)	Sujet + have/has + not + participe passé	Have/Has + sujet + participe passé
I have worked a lot today.	I have not (haven't) finished yet.	Have you ever taken antibiotics?

GRAMMAR

Present perfect progressif

• Emploi

– Pour parler d'actions commencées dans le passé mais qui continuent dans le présent ou qui viennent de se terminer. L'accent est mis :

. Soit sur la durée de l'action : He has been working all week.

. Soit sur le résultat : "You look tired. – Yes, I've been working all night".

– Avec for et since quand ils signifient « depuis » (voir p. 87).

• Construction

Forme affirmative	Forme négative	Forme interrogative
Sujet + have/has + been + verbe en -ing	Sujet + have/has + not + been + verbe en -ing	have/has + sujet + been + verbe en -ing
He has been waiting for a long time.	He has not (hasn't) been waiting long.	Has he been waiting long?

Exercice 1

Réponse p. 75

Test rapide pour réviser les verbes irréguliers. Complétez le tableau ci-dessous.

Infinitif	Preterit	Present perfect
To be	was/were	I have been
To break	....	....
To bring	....	....
To come	....	....
To cut	....	....
To do	....	....
To drink	....	....
To eat	....	....
To feel	....	....
To find	....	....
To give	....	....

Exercice 2

Réponse p. 75

Complétez les phrases suivantes en employant le present perfect.

1. They (*meet*) .... recently .... my daughter.
2. She (*do*) .... just .... a dressing.
3. He (*break*) .... never .... his leg.
4. They (*be*) .... already .... to the psychiatric ward.
5. She (*finish*) .... not .... yet.

Travaillez à deux : Preterit ou present perfect

Réponse p. 75

A. est médecin, B. est son patient.

Écrivez sous forme de dialogue les informations ci-dessous ; puis inversez les rôles.

1. Avez-vous déjà subi un test de dépistage ?	Sa réponse est : oui.
2. Quand l'avez-vous subi pour la dernière fois ?	Sa réponse est : il y a trois mois.
3. Quand avez-vous remarqué des symptômes ?	Sa réponse est : l'hiver dernier.
4. Depuis combien de temps toussez-vous ?	Sa réponse est : deux semaines.
5. Avez-vous pris des médicaments le mois dernier ?	Sa réponse est : oui.

1. **A.** Doctor: ....
   B. Patient: ....
2. **A.** Doctor: ....
   B. Patient: ....
3. **A.** Doctor: ....
   B. Patient: ....
4. **A.** Doctor: ....
   B. Patient: ....
5. **A.** Doctor: ....
   B. Patient: ....

Piste 21 Exercice 3

Réponse p. 75

Écoutez, puis répétez.

Complétez la légende à l'aide des mots suivants :

- shaving cream
- temperature chart
- washbasin
- comb
- toothbrush
- bed head
- towel
- blanket
- mattress
- shampoo
- razor
- soap
- sheet
- toothpaste
- drawer

Personal hygiene

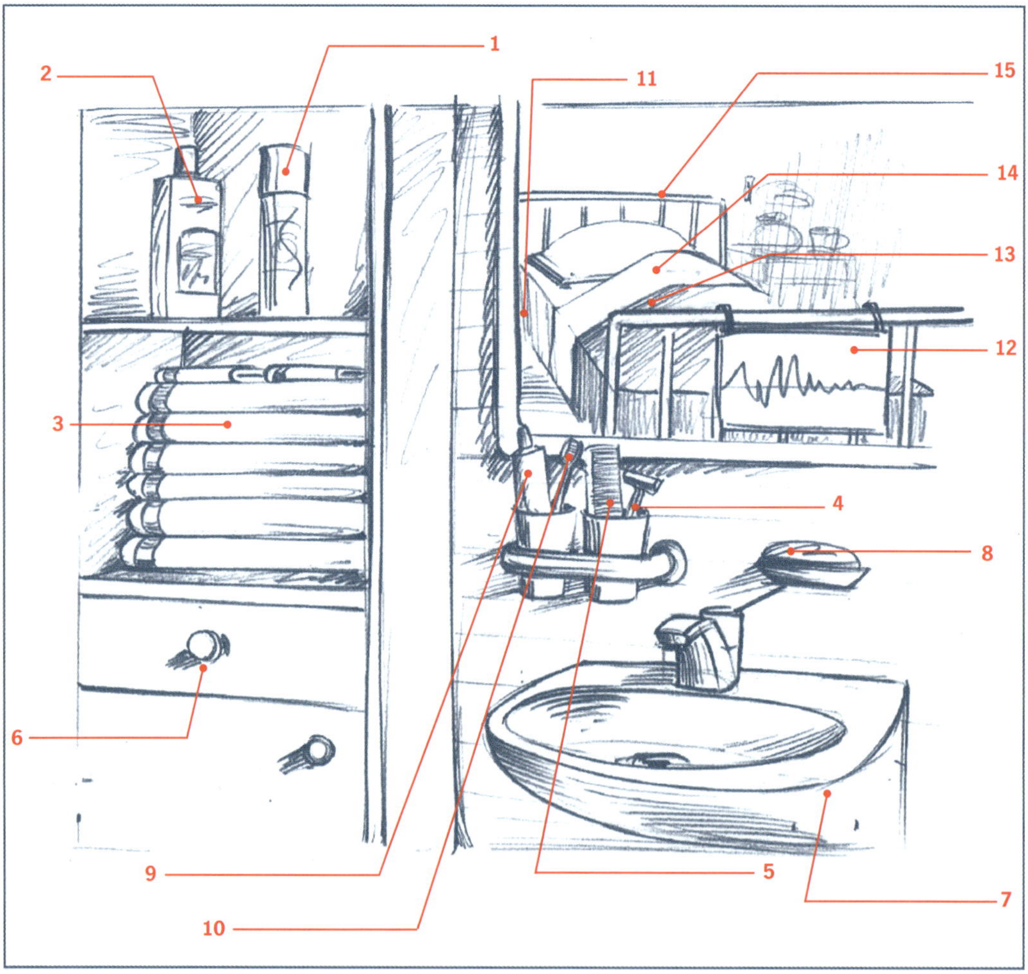

https://www.lienmini.fr/angsoin09

Exercice 4 : Advising a patient with a plaster cast

Piste 22

Traduction pp. 209-210
Réponse p. 75

Écoutez le dialogue.

Complétez la conversation entre le médecin et sa patiente à l'aide des phrases suivantes :

- ... if there is an unusual smell
- Is the plaster too tight*?
- ... your fibula were put back together again
- ... you must keep it dry.
- The plaster will take...

Doctor I had to* reduce your fracture before putting your plaster on.

Patient What does "reduce" mean, please Doctor?

Doctor The two parts of **(1)** ....

Patient Oh, I see.

Doctor **(2)** ....

Patient No, it's all right.

Doctor I must give you some advice before you leave the hospital. **(3)** .... 48 hours to dry*. So, **(4)** ....

Patient Of course. Can I walk?

Doctor You can walk with crutches*. But let me know immediately if there is a loss of feeling or if your foot becomes cold.

Patient All right, I understand.

Doctor I have one more piece of advice. You must tell me at once* **(5)** ....

To help you

- **tight:** serré
- **I had to:** j'ai dû
- **to dry:** sécher
- **crutches:** cannes anglaises
- **at once:** immédiatement

Exercice 5

Piste 23

Réponse p. 75

Écoutez et complétez les phrases.

1. Keep your arm raised on a pillow ....

2. Don't get your plaster cast wet. This will weaken it ....

3. You can use a plastic bag to cover up the cast ....

4. Remove the bag as soon as you can, ...

UNIT 5

GRAMMAR

Exprimer la quantité : some/any (du, de la, des, en)

• Some

On emploie some :
- dans une phrase affirmative : I would like some tea.
- dans une phrase interrogative quand on offre quelque chose : Would you like some tea?

• Any

On emploie any :
- dans une phrase négative : There isn't any tea (There is no tea).
- dans une phrase interrogative quand on ne sait pas s'il y en a : Have you got any brothers? – No, I haven't/ No, I haven't got any.
- après without, never, hardly :
  . The patient tried to walk without any help.
  . There are hardly any patients left in the waiting-room.
- dans une phrase affirmative avec anybody (n'importe qui), anything (n'importe quoi), anywhere (n'importe où) : I can sleep anywhere.

Exercice 6

Réponse p. 75

Complétez les phrases à l'aide de *any, some, no*.

1. There aren't .... anti-inflammatory drugs left.
2. Is there .... body here?
3. .... vaccines must be kept under refrigeration.
4. Have you got .... compresses? No, I haven't. Could you bring me ...., please?
5. She did not want to take .... medication.
6. She went to the lab but there was .... body there.

Exercice 7

Réponse p. 76

Complétez avec *dead, death* ou *to die* (conjugué au bon temps).

Rappels :
- **He is dead:** *Il est mort*. C'est un constat.
- **He died last year:** *Il est mort l'année dernière. Il mourut.* Verbe mourir conjugué au passé.
- **Death:** *la mort.*

1. Three AIDS patients .... last week.
2. Her .... was a shock to all her friends.
3. Every year, many smokers .... from lung cancer.
4. Most of the people I know fear ....
5. Mr da Silva in Room 104 is .... He .... at 2 o'clock this morning.
6. She .... of breast cancer two weeks ago.

Piste 24

Exercice 8

Réponse p. 76

Écoutez, puis répétez.
Complétez la légende avec les mots suivants :

- phalanges
- sacrum
- pelvis
- tibia/shin
- fibula
- patella
- femur
- cubitus
- radius
- humerus
- sternum
- ribs
- clavicle
- skull
- vertebral column/spine
- mandible/jaw

The skeleton

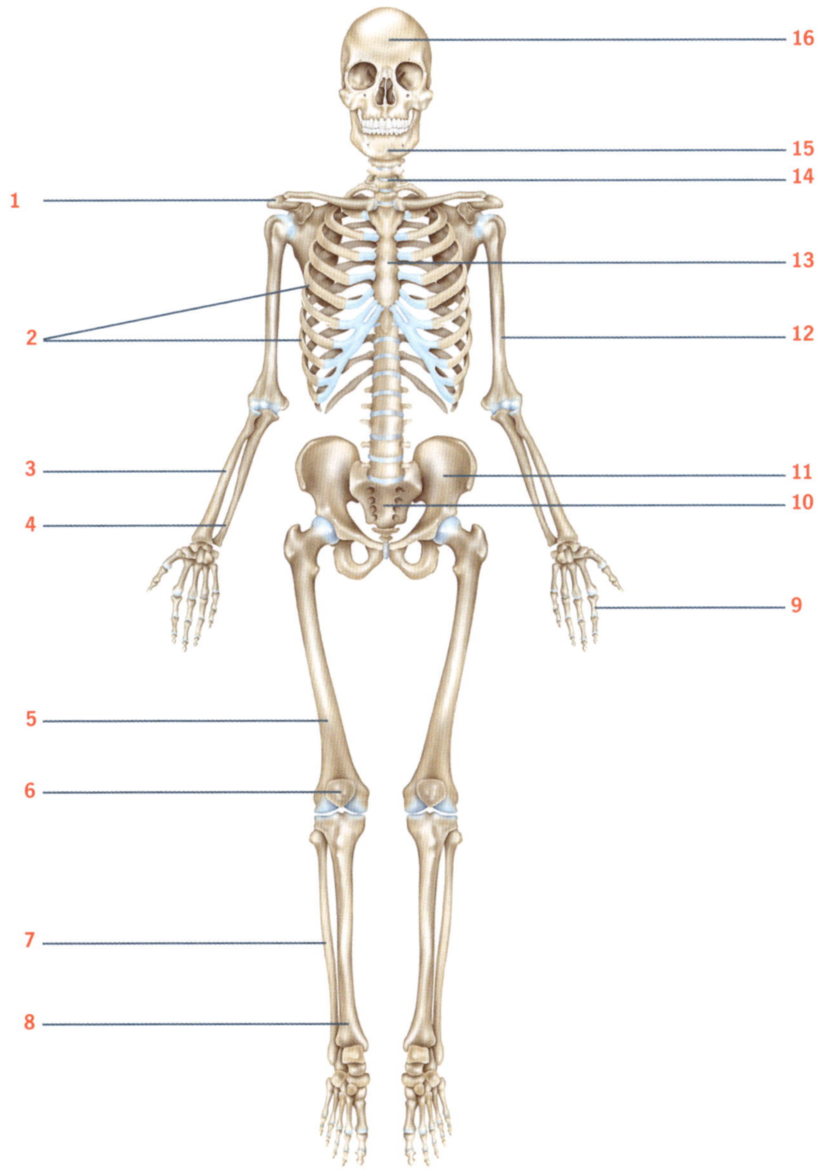

https://www.lienmini.fr/angsoin10

5 UNIT

Travaillez à deux : Culture

"Each person is culturally unique."

A.: You are a nurse.
Ask **B** questions about his/her culture (beliefs, behaviours, habits, language, rituals, religious ceremonies).

B.: You are a foreign patient (from Africa, or Asia, or South America...).

Exercice 9 : Testez-vous !

Réponse p. 76

Traduisez en anglais.

1. Pourriez-vous inspirer puis expirer la bouche ouverte, s'il vous plaît ? ....

2. Est-ce que c'est douloureux quand j'appuie ici ? ....

3. Pourriez-vous vous retourner puis lever votre bras, s'il vous plaît ? ....

4. Elle vient d'appliquer de la pommade pour éviter les escarres. ....

5. Avez-vous déjà fait son pansement ? Non, pas encore. ....

6. Une prise de sang doit être faite régulièrement quand une personne est sous anticoagulants.

7. Il ne reste plus d'anti-inflammatoires dans le tiroir. ....

Exercice 10 : Healthcare assistant education

Réponse p. 76

How to give a bed bath

Cochez la (les) bonne(s) affirmation(s).

	True	False
1. Bed baths are used to bathe people who are are bedridden* or unable to bathe on their own* due to health reasons.		
2. Giving a bed bath involves* washing and rinsing the entire body one part at a time while the patient stays in bed.		
3. It is important to gather* all the supplies needed before you begin so you do not have to leave the patient unattended.		
4. A good bed bath will leave the person feeling clean and comfortable.		
5. You need two washbowls* with cold water.		

To help you

- **bedridden:** grabattaire
- **on their own:** tout seuls
- **to involve:** impliquer, signifier
- **to gather:** rassembler
- **unattended:** sans surveillance
- **washbowl:** cuvette pour la toilette

https://www.lienmini.fr/angsoinq5a

Verbs quiz

Réponse p. 76

Complétez chaque affirmation avec le verbe correct.

1. The GP .... up at 6.00 every morning to go to hospital.
a) gets **b)** got **c)** has got **d)** get

2. She always .... breakfast in her bedroom.
a) takes **b)** does **c)** eats **d)** has

3. He .... a screening test last week.
a) has had **b)** have **c)** had **d)** has

4. May I .... your stetoscope, I've forgotten mine ?
a) take **b)** put **c)** borrow **d)** lend

5. I .... a medical documentary on TV last night.
a) looked at **b)** read **c)** watched **d)** heard

https://www.lienmini.fr/angsoinq5b

Vocabulary quiz

Réponse p. 76

Complétez chaque affirmation avec le terme correct.

1. Breathe in and out with your .... open.
a) nose **b)** ear **c)** mouth **d)** eye

2. A .... helps patients to give them a bedbath.
a) nurse **b)** specialist **c)** surgeon **d)** healthcare assistant

3. To have a .... you need shampoo, soap and a towel.
a) shave **b)** shower **c)** meal **d)** cold

4. You rub on some ointment to prevent ....
a) coughing **b)** bedsores **c)** headache **d)** the flu

5. The human .... consists of 206 bones.
a) organs **b)** skull **c)** skeleton **d)** vertebral column/spine

Medical Vocabulary: unit 5

- **to breathe out:** expirer
- **to cough:** tousser
- **crutches:** cannes anglaises
- **screening test:** test de dépistage
- **pelvis (anat.):** bassin
- **fibula:** péroné
- **skull:** crâne
- **in a sling:** en écharpe

Let's discuss!

Palliative care

What do you know about palliative care?
Is it a field of nursing in which you would like to work? Why or why not?

Corrigés

Exercice 1

Infinitif	Preterit	Present Perfect
To be	was/were	I have been
To break	broke	I have broken
To bring	brought	I have brought
To come	came	I have come
To cut	cut	I have cut
To do	did	I have done
To drink	drank	I have drunk
To eat	ate	I have eaten
To feel	felt	I have felt
To find	found	I have found
To give	gave	I have given

Exercice 2

1. They **have** recently **met** my daughter.
2. She **has** just **done** a dressing.
3. He **has** never **broken** his leg.
4. They **have** already **been** to the psychiatric ward.
5. She **has** not **finished** yet.

Travaillez à deux

1. **Doctor:** Have you ever had a screening test?
Patient: Yes, I have.
2. **Doctor:** When did you last have one?
Patient: I (last) had one three months ago.
3. **Doctor:** When did you notice the symptoms?
Patient: I noticed them last winter.
4. **Doctor:** How long have you had a cough?/ How long have you been coughing?
Patient: I've had a cough for two weeks.
5. **Doctor:** Did you take any medication last month?
Patient: Yes, I did.

Exercice 3

1. shaving cream
2. shampoo
3. towel
4. razor
5. comb
6. drawer
7. washbasin
8. soap
9. toothpaste
10. toothbrush
11. mattress
12. temperature chart
13. blanket
14. sheet
15. bed head

Exercice 4

1. ... your fibula were put together again.
2. Is the plaster too tight?
3. The plaster will take ....
4. ... you must keep it dry.
5. if there is an unusual smell.

Exercice 5

1. Keep your arm raised on a pillow **for the first 12 hours and rest**.
2. Don't get your plaster cast wet. This will weaken it **and the bone won't be properly supported**.
3. You can use a plastic bag to cover up the cast **when you have a bath or shower**.
4. Remove the bag as soon as you can, **to avoid sweating**.

Exercice 6

1. There aren't **any** anti-inflammatory drugs left.
2. Is there **any**body here?
3. **Some** vaccines must be kept under refrigeration.
4. Have you got **any** compresses? No, I haven't. Could you bring me **some**, please?
5. She did not want to take **any** medication.
6. She went to the lab but there was **no**body there.

Corrigés

Exercice 7

1. Three AIDS patients **died** last week.
2. Her **death** was a shock to all her friends.
3. Every year, many smokers **die** from lung cancer.
4. Most of the people I know fear **death**.
5. Mr da Silva in Room 104 is **dead**. He **died** at 2 o'clock this morning.
6. She **died** of breast cancer two weeks ago.

Exercice 8

1. clavicle
2. ribs
3. radius
4. cubitus
5. femur
6. patella
7. fibula
8. tibia/shin
9. phalanges
10. sacrum
11. pelvis
12. humerus
13. sternum
14. vertebral column/spine
15. mandible/jaw
16. skull

Exercice 9 : Testez-vous !

1. Could you breathe in and out with your mouth open, please?
2. Does it hurt when I press here?
3. Could you turn round and lift your arm please?
4. She has just rubbed on some ointment to prevent bedsores.
5. Have you already dressed his/her wound? No, not yet.
6. A blood test must be done regularly when a person takes anticoagulants.
7. There are no anti-inflammatories left in the drawer./There aren't any anti-inflammatories left in the drawer.

Exercice 10

1. True
2. True
3. True
4. True
5. False

Verbs quiz

1. gets
2. has
3. had
4. borrow
5. watched

Vocabulary quiz

1. mouth
2. healthcare assistant
3. shower
4. bedsores
5. skeleton

UNIT 6

UNIT 6 Taking a blood sample and changing a drip*

Toutes les pistes audio de l'unité à télécharger ici
https://www.lienmini.fr/angsoinu6

Piste 25

Dialogue between Mr Brown and the nurse, and Mrs Jones and the nurse

Traduction p. 210

Listen to the dialogue. After his operation, Mr Brown suffered from heart complications: a pulmonary embolism. He is under medical supervision*. A nurse is coming to take a blood sample*.

Nurse Good morning Mr Brown. How are you today?
Mr Brown So, so*. I didn't sleep very well last night.
Nurse Why didn't you call the nurse on duty*?
Mr Brown Well, I didn't dare*... Could you tell me why I'm still on a drip*?
Nurse Because we need to treat you with anticoagulants and other drugs intravenously.
Mr Brown Oh, I see.
Nurse I have to take a blood sample now.
Mr Brown But you've only just taken one.
Nurse Yes, I know. But because you're taking anticoagulants we have to do a blood test regularly to check if the treatment is working. If you feel any pain when the needle goes in, tell me please.
Mr Brown No, it's all right. I'm used to it* now!

In the bedroom opposite, a male nurse is changing a drip.

Nurse Good morning, Mrs Jones.
Mrs Jones Good morning.
Nurse Now, I'm going to change your drip because it doesn't function very well.
Mrs Jones What is that?
Nurse It's a tourniquet*. We use it so that we can see your vein more clearly. I'm going to put the needle in. Don't worry. It may hurt a little.
Mrs Jones But why am I still on a drip?
Nurse Because you've had an operation. Have you passed wind* recently?
Mrs Jones No, not yet.
Nurse So, your digestive system is stilla little slow. Please try to keep your arm still while* I'm changing your drip.
Mrs Jones Oh, sorry...
Nurse It's all right*. I'll change your bag every six hours. See you later.

To help you

- **to change a drip:** changer une perfusion
- **under medical supervision:** sous surveillance médicale
- **to take a blood sample:** faire une prise de sang
- **so, so:** comme ci, comme ça
- **the nurse on duty:** l'infirmière de garde
- **to dare:** oser
- **I'm still on a drip:** je suis encore sous perfusion
- **I'm used to it:** j'y suis habitué
- **tourniquet:** garrot
- **to pass/to have wind:** avoir des gaz
- **still:** immobile
- **while:** pendant que
- **it's all right:** ce n'est pas grave (ici)

Questions sur le dialogue

1. Why is Mr Brown still on a drip? ....

2. Why does the nurse regularly take a blood sample? ....

3. Is Mr Brown very sensitive to the needle? Why or why not? ....

4. What is a tourniquet for? ....

5. How can the nurse tell Mrs Jones' digestive system is still a little slow? ....

6. How often will the nurse change the bag? ....

UNIT 6

GRAMMAR

Past continuous

• Emploi

On utilise le past continuous pour parler d'une action passée qui se déroule en même temps qu'une autre. Il correspond souvent à l'imparfait français. On peut également le remplacer par « j'étais en train de ».

• Construction

Forme affirmative	Sujet + auxiliaire was/were + verbe à la forme -ing	She was reading the patient's medical record when I arrived.
Forme négative	Sujet + auxiliaire was/were + not + verbe à la forme -ing	She was not (wasn't) talking to the nurse when I came in.
Forme interrogative	Auxiliaire was/were + sujet + verbe à la forme -ing	What were you doing last night at 10:00?

Exercice 1

Réponse p. 91

Voici des actions qui se sont déroulées au moment où une sonnette s'est déclenchée. Que faisait chaque personne à cet instant ?

Ex.: When the bell rang David (*have*) a shower.
When the bell rang David ***was having*** a shower.

When the bell rang:

1. Denis (*write*) a medical report: ....
2. Carole and Lucy (*make*) a bed: ....
3. Anne (*shave*) a patient: ....
4. Tristan (*answer*) the phone: ....
5. Marie (*take*) a blood sample: ....

Travaillez à deux

Demandez à votre partenaire ce que faisaient ses collègues hier quand il/elle est arrivé(e) dans son service.

Ex.:

A. What was Marie doing when you entered the unit/ward?
B. When I entered the unit she was changing a drip.

Puis, inversez les rôles.

Exercice 2

Réponse p. 91

Complétez avec le prétérit simple ou le prétérit progressif continu (past continuous).

1. She .... (*put on*) a plaster when the senior nurse .... (*call*) her.
2. He .... (*remove*) a drain when the doctor .... (*arrive*).
3. When the bell .... (*ring*), she .... (*insert*) a catheter.
4. When she .... (*phone*) me, I .... (*take*) my cough syrup.
5. He .... (*check for*) her vital signs, when the surgeon .... (*ask*) him to come at once.
6. She .... (*take*) her temperature whereas I .... (*do*) a dressing in room 25.

Piste 26

Exercice 3

Réponse p. 91

Écoutez, puis répétez.
Complétez la légende à l'aide des mots suivants :

- drops
- tablet
- capsule
- syrup
- skin patch
- suppository
- ointment

Drugs/medicines/medication[1]

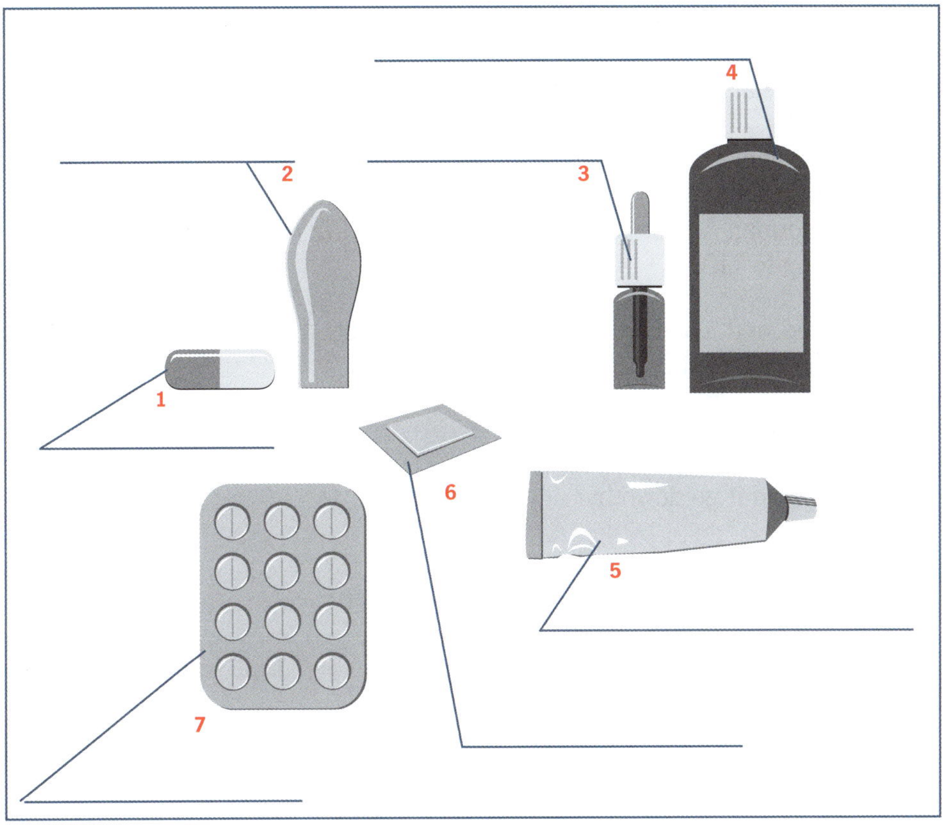

© C.K.

https://www.lienmini.fr/angsoin11

Measurement units

1 teaspoon = 5 ml	1 tablespoon = 15 ml	standard catheter = 1 ml	syringe = 15 drops

1. – *Medicine tends to refer to liquid medication.*
   – *Medication is a more generic term.*

Piste 27

Exercice 4 : Talking about blood pressure, temperature and pulse

Traduction p. 211
Réponse p. 91

Écoutez le dialogue puis complétez la conversation entre le médecin et l'infirmière. Utilisez les phrases suivantes :

- I took it half an hour ago
- ... she had a lot of visitors this afternoon.
- It fell by two points (degrees)
- has increased

Doctor Now, how is Mrs Weeks' blood pressure today?

Nurse It was steady at 150/80[1] until this morning. But it went up an hour ago. Maybe it's because **(1)** ....
But everything is all right now. As for her temperature, it rose slightly this morning, but now it's steady. **(2)** .... It was back to normal. And as for Mr Jones, his pulse **(3)** ....
It's now up to 110.

Doctor Well, I'll go and see him immediately. But before that, tell me about Mr Joyce's temperature. It went up to 41 °C last night.

Nurse It went down sharply this morning.

Doctor How much did it go down by?

Nurse **(4)** .... but now it's stable.

---

1. Blood pressure is expressed differently in English-speaking countries: France - 15/8 becomes 150/80 in the UK (we multiply the value by 10).

Exercice 5

Réponse p. 91

Inscrivez sous les trois courbes les verbes qui leur correspondent.

- to go up
- to remain steady
- to stay the same
- to remain constant
- to rise
- to fall
- to decrease
- to increase
- to go down

How to describe a graph or temperature curve

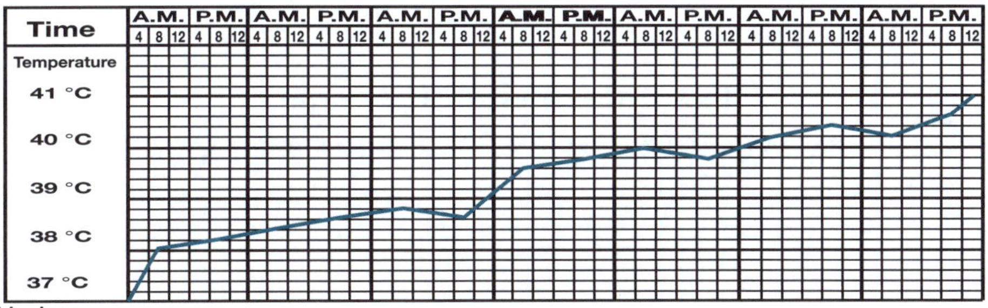

Verbs: ....

....

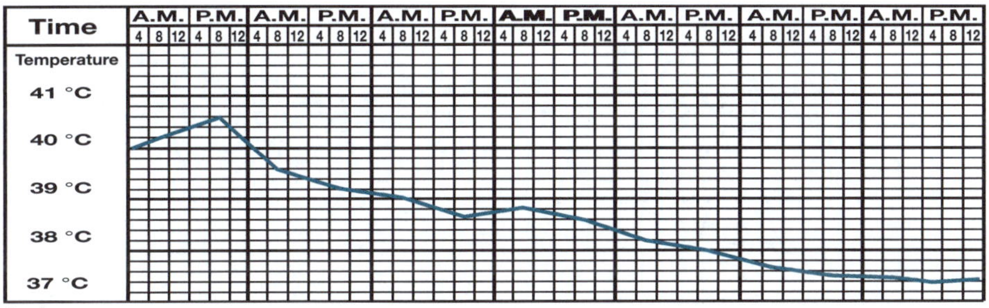

Verbs: ....

....

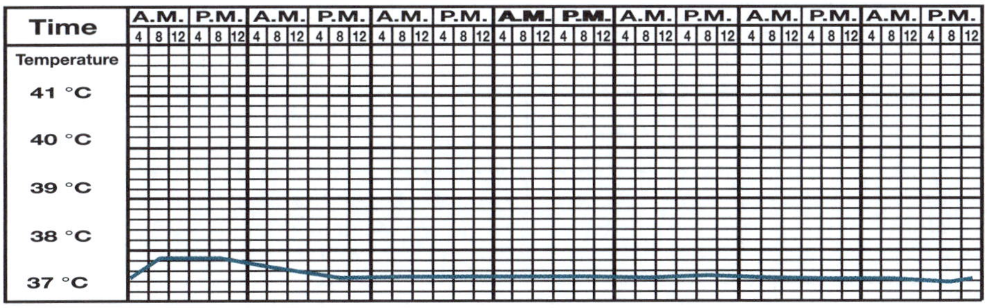

Verbs: ....

....

Travaillez à deux

Dessinez sur la feuille ci-dessous la courbe de température d'un patient sur plusieurs jours, puis faites-en un commentaire oral à votre partenaire, en vous aidant des verbes de la page précédente et de la liste ci-dessous.

Faites de même pour les autres paramètres (pulse and blood pressure).

- slightly: légèrement
- steadily: régulièrement
- sharply: brusquement
- dangerously: gravement, sérieusement
- encouragingly: d'une manière encourageante
- up to: jusqu'à
- until now: jusqu'à présent

Example of vital signs chart

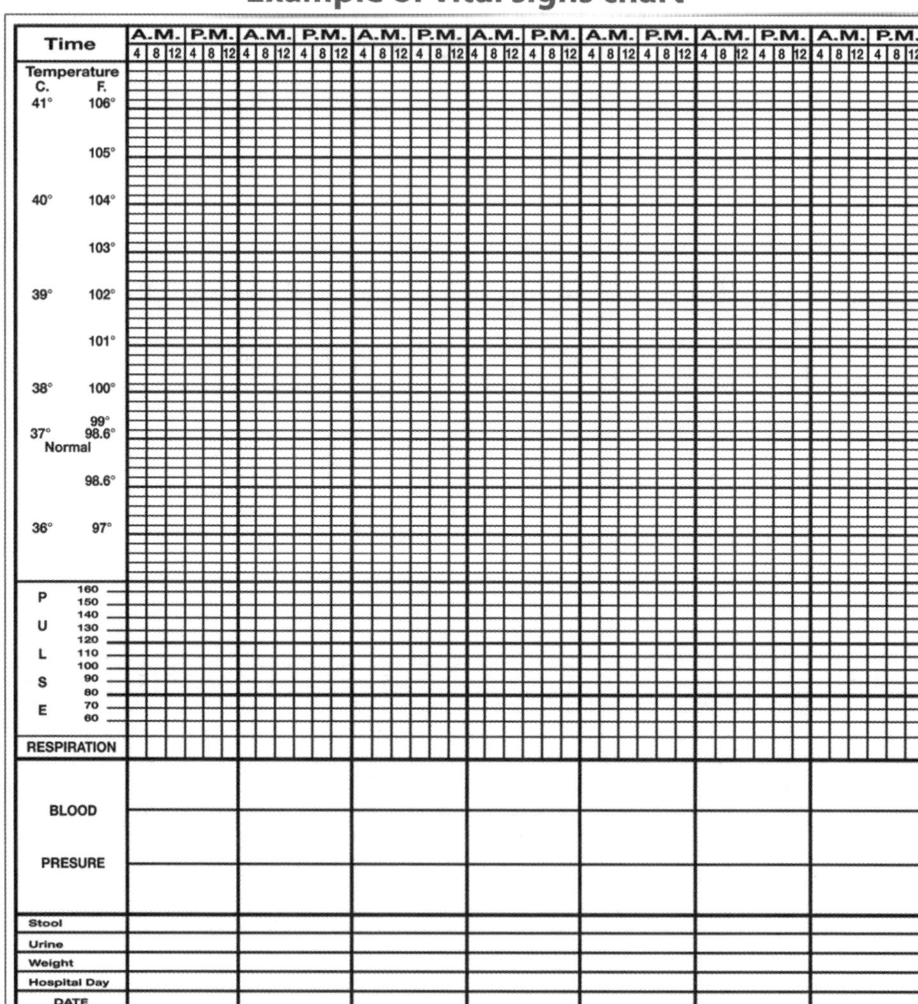

Measurement units - Temperature

°C = Celsius

°F = Fahrenheit

°C = [(°F − 32) × 5]/9

°F = [(9 × °C)/5] + 32

Ex. : 36 °C = 96.8 °F   37 °C = 98.6 °F   38 °C = 100 °F   39 °C = 102 °F

Piste 28

Exercice 6

Réponse p. 91

Écoutez, puis répétez.

Complétez la légende avec les mots suivants :

- oesophagus/gullet
- anus
- colon
- liver
- stomach
- small intestine
- pancreas
- gall-bladder

Digestive system

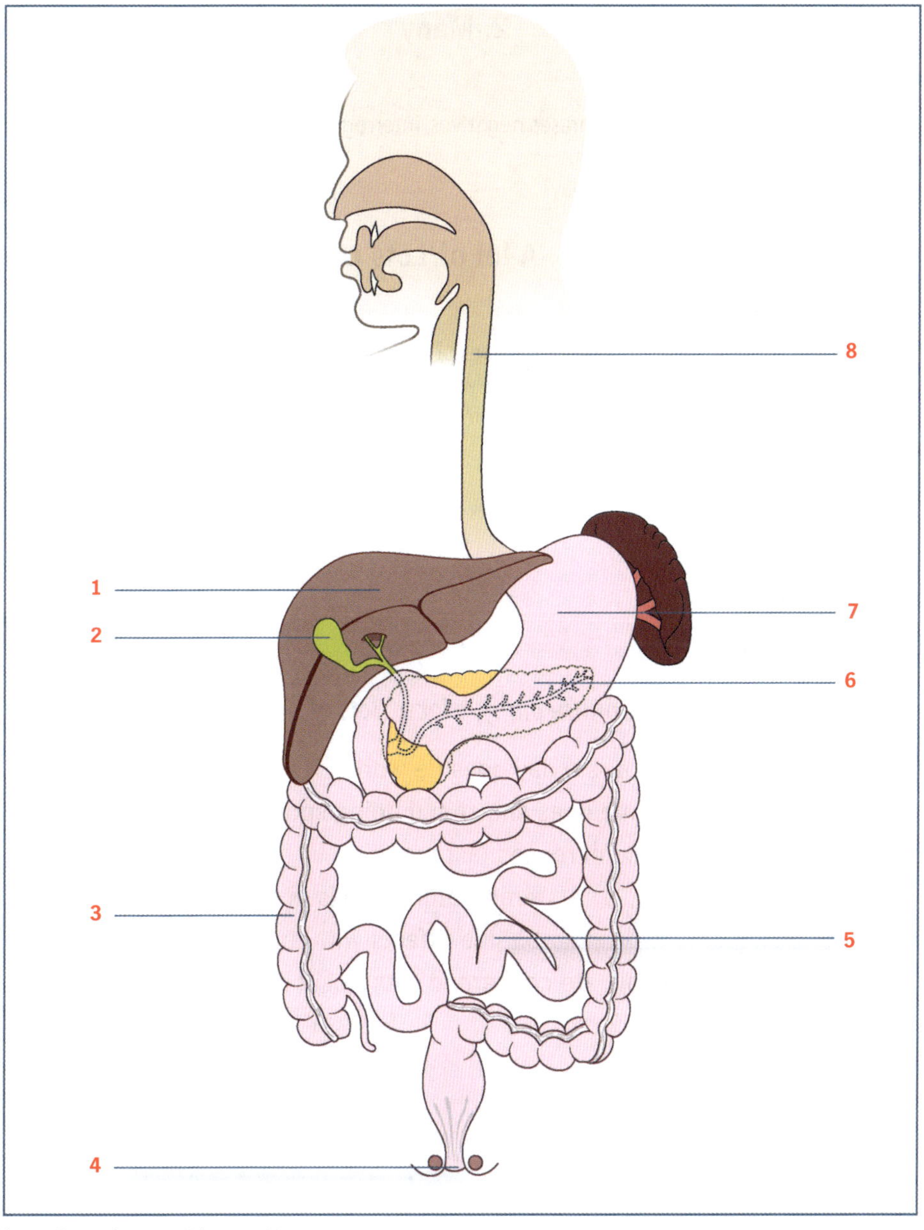

© S.M.

https://www.lienmini.fr/angsoin12

6 UNIT

GRAMMAR

Exprimer la quantité : beaucoup
Much/many/a lot of/lots of

1. Much

• ***Quand l'emploie-t-on ?***

– Après un nom au singulier, dans les phrases négatives, interrogatives et affirmatives :
. The intern didn't have much time to see the patient.
. Did you take much cough syrup last night?

2. Many

• ***Quand l'emploie-t-on ?***

– Après un nom au pluriel, dans les phrases négatives, interrogatives et affirmatives :
. There aren't many skin-patches left.
. Did you change many drips yesterday?

3. A lot of/Lots of

• ***Quand l'emploie-t-on ?***

– Après un nom au singulier ou au pluriel, dans les phrases affirmatives :
. The senioonr nurse has a lot of meetings this week.
. She took a lot of cough syrup yesterday evening.

Exercice 7

Réponse p. 91

Complétez les phrases à l'aide de *much, many, a lot of, lots of.*

1. How .... hours a day does he work?
2. How .... time does she spend doing sport?
3. I had .... conferences last month.
4. There weren't .... temperature charts in the cupboard.
5. There will not be .... side-effects with this medication.
6. .... hospitals are concerned with nosocomial infections.

GRAMMAR

Exprimer la quantité : peu
A few/a little/few/little

A few ***Quelques*** Quand l'emploie-t-on ? Devant un pluriel : – He has a few friends.	***A little*** ***Un peu (de)*** Quand l'emploie-t-on ? Devant un singulier : – May I have a little water, please?
Few ***Peu (de)*** Quand l'emploie-t-on ? Devant un pluriel : – There were few infections on this ward.	***Little*** ***Peu (de)*** Quand l'emploie-t-on ? Devant un singulier : – He spent little time in Dublin.

Exercice 8

Réponse p. 91

Complétez les phrases à l'aide de *a little, little, a few, few.*

1. In the past ten years, there have been .... outbreaks of measles in Africa.
2. White rice contains .... nutritional value.
3. Very .... people are not able to see the difference between red and green.
4. .... people were reading magazines in the waiting-room.
5. Hurry up! We have .... time left.
6. His salary is low: he earns very .... money.
7. This drug had .... side-effects.
8. You don't have to hurry: we have .... time left.
9. She was disappointed because she had .... visitors.
10. He was recovering .... by ....

Exercice 9 : Testez-vous !

Réponse p. 92

Traduisez en anglais.

1. Quand il est arrivé dans la chambre, elle posait une perfusion. ....

2. Je lui donnais des gélules quand le médecin m'a demandé sa feuille de température. .....

3. Prenez vingt gouttes avant les repas et deux cachets avant de vous coucher. ....

4. Quel traitement suivez-vous actuellement ? Vous ne devez pas l'arrêter brusquement. ....

5. Sa tension a chuté sérieusement hier soir. ....

6. Sa température a augmenté brusquement plusieurs fois hier. ....

7. Son pouls s'est stabilisé. ....

Exercice 10 : Patient education

Réponse p. 92

Vital signs

Cochez la (les) bonne(s) affirmation(s).

	True	False
1. Body temperature can be taken orally (by mouth), rectally, axillary (under the arm), by ear, by skin.		
2. The pulse rate is a measurement of the heart rate, or the number of times the heart beats per minute		
3. The respiration rate (rate of breathing) is the number of breaths a person takes per minute.		
4. Respiration rates may not increase with fever, illness, and with other medical conditions.		
5. Blood pressure (measured with a blood pressure cuff* and stethoscope by a nurse) is the force of the blood pushing against the artery walls.		

To help you

- **blood pressure cuff:** brassard de tensiomètre

https://www.lienmini.fr/angsoinq6a

Vocabulary quiz: Drugs and medicines

Réponse p. 92

Complétez chaque définition avec le terme correct.

1. A .... is a small round solid piece of medicine inside that you swallow.
a) syrup **b)** suppository **c)** tablet **d)** vial*

2. A small container which has measured amount of a medicine inside and which dissolves when you swallow it is called a ....
a) drop **b)** capsule **c)** syrup **d)** patch

3. An .... is a small container containing drug thas is used for an injection.
a) patch **b)** ampoule **c)** capsule **d)** tablet

4. A phial* or a .... is a small container containing drug that you swallow.
a) patch **b)** tablet **c)** vial **d)** ointment

5. To prevent bedsores you rub some .... on the skin.
a) syrup **b)** ether **c)** ointment **d)** patch

https://www.lienmini.fr/angsoinq6b

Human body quiz

Réponse p. 92

Complétez chaque affirmation avec le terme correct.

1. My daughter's little .... was lost in a car accident.
a) thumb **b)** foot **c)** toe **d)** arm

2. I'll put a cool cloth on your .... to get your fever down.
a) skin **b)** forehead **c)** hand **d)** leg

3. Another word for joint is ....
a) bone **b)** organ **c)** muscle **d)** articulation

4. He had a heart attack last week because of his .... problem.
a) kidney **b)** liver **c)** cardiac **d)** lung

5. He may never walk again because his .... is seriously injured.
a) spine **b)** gall-bladder **c)** stomach **d)** eye

To help you

- **vial:** ampoule
- **phial :** flacon, ampoule

UNIT 6

Medical Vocabulary: unit 6

- **blood sample:** prise de sang
- **drip:** perfusion
- **tourniquet:** garrot
- **liver:** foie
- **gall-bladder:** vésicule biliaire
- **to remove a drain:** retirer un drain
- **to insert a catheter:** poser un cathéter
- **ointment:** pommade
- **drops:** gouttes
- **temperature curve/chart:** courbe/feuille de température

Let's discuss!

Administering medication

Little Sam's death: nurse indicted*.

Last Wednesday a nurse admitted inserting a drip of magnesium chloride by mistake into three-year-old Sam, causing his death. In her defence, she claimed the flask containing the magnesium chloride was not located in the usual place.
She was indicted for manslaughter* and has been put on probation*.

Drug labelling*.

The Minister of Health recently released* a circular calling for all injectable drug labels to be more legible, particularly magnesium chloride which was responsible for Sam's death. "The objective of this is to minimize the risk of therapeutic error".

What's your opinion on this subject?

To help you

- **to be indicted:** être mis en examen
- **manslaughter:** homicide involontaire
- **to be put on probation:** être placé sous contrôle judiciaire
- **labelling:** étiquetage
- **to release:** faire paraître

Exercice 1

When the alarm rang:

1. Denis **was writing** a medical report.
2. Carole and Lucy **were making** a bed.
3. Anne **was shaving** a patient.
4. Tristan **was answering** the phone.
5. Marie **was taking** a blood sample.

Exercice 2

1. She **was putting** on a plaster when the senior nurse **called** her.
2. He **was removing** the drain when the doctor **arrived**.
3. When the bell **rang**, she **was inserting** a catheter.
4. When she **phoned** me, I **was taking** my syrup.
5. He **was checking** for her vital signs, when the surgeon **asked** him to come at once.
6. She **was taking** her temperature whereas I **was doing** a dressing in room 25.

Exercice 3

1. capsule
2. suppository
3. drops
4. syrup
5. ointment
6. skin patch
7. tablet

Exercice 4

1. ... she had a lot of visitors this afternoon.
2. I took it half an hour ago.
3. ... has increased.
4. It fell by two degrees (points).

Exercice 5

1. to go up/to rise/to increase.
2. to decrease/to fall/to go down.
3. to remain constant/to remain steady/to stay the same.

Exercice 6

1. liver
2. gall-bladder
3. colon
4. anus
5. small intestine
6. pancreas
7. stomach
8. oesophagus/gullet

Exercice 7

1. How **many** hours a day does he work?
2. How **much** time does she spend doing sport?
3. I had **many** conferences last month.
4. There weren't **many** temperature charts in the cupboard.
5. There will not be **many** side-effects with this medication.
6. **A lot of/lots of/many** hospitals are concerned with nosocomial infections.

Exercice 8

1. In the past ten years, there have been **few/a few** outbreaks of measles in Africa.
2. White rice contains **little** nutritional value.
3. Very **few** people are not able to see the difference between red and green.
4. **A few** people were reading magazines in the waiting-room.
5. Hurry up! We have **little** time left.
6. His salary is low: he earns very **little** money.
7. This drug had **few/a few** side-effects.
8. You don't have to hurry: we have **a little** time left.
9. She was disappointed because she had **few** visitors.
10. He was recovering **little** by **little**.

Corrigés

Exercice 9 : Testez-vous !

1. When he came into the room, she was putting up a drip.
2. I was giving him/her capsules when the doctor asked me for his/her temperature chart.
3. Take twenty drops before meals and two tablets before going to bed.
4. Which medication/treatment are you on currently/at the moment? You mustn't stop it abruptly.
5. His/her blood pressure decreased/went down dangerously last night.
6. His/her temperature increased/went up/rose sharply several times yesterday.
7. His/her pulse has remained steady/constant.

Exercice 10

1. True
2. True
3. True
4. False
5. True

Vocabulary quiz: Drugs and medicines

1. tablet
2. capsule
3. ampoule
4. vial
5. ointment

Human body quiz

1. toe
2. forehead
3. articulation
4. cardiac
5. spine

UNIT 7

UNIT 7

Reassuring the patient

Toutes les pistes audio de l'unité à télécharger ici
https://www.lienmini.fr/angsoinu7

Piste 29

Dialogue between Mr Brown and the nurse

Traduction p. 211

Listen to the dialogue. Because of his heart complications, Mr Brown's morale has been low since this morning. The nurse is doing her best to reassure him and to make him feel better.

Nurse Good morning, Mr Brown.

Mr Brown Good morning.

Nurse How are you today?

Mr Brown Not so good. I've been here for two weeks and I'm not getting any better.

Nurse Yes, I know but that's normal after a pulmonary embolism. Everything will be all right now. You're getting the right treatment.

Mr Brown Yes, but my back was hurting a lot during the night.

Nurse I'm sorry to hear that, but you've been in bed for a long time*.

Mr Brown Yes... well... I miss my family*. My son went back to England last week, and I wonder if I'll ever see my grandchildren again...

Nurse Please, don't worry. I suppose it's more difficult to be ill in a foreign country, but your wife visits you everyday, doesn't she?

Mr Brown Yes, that's true. But you know it's hard to tell her how I'm feeling, sometimes.

Nurse Don't hesitate to tell me if there is something bothering you*. I'm sorry, I have to go now, but I'll come back this afternoon and we'll have another chat. And don't forget: the important thing is to keep up your morale*.

Mr Brown Well, thank you for your help. See you this afternoon.

To help you

- **for a long time:** depuis longtemps
- **I miss my family:** ma famille me manque
- **to bother:** tracasser/préoccuper
- **to keep up your morale:** garder le moral

Questions sur le dialogue

1. Why has Mr Brown been feeling down? ....

2. How long has he been in hospital? ....

3. Why has he got backache? ....

4. What does he worry about? ....

5. Why is it more difficult to be ill in a foreign country? ....

6. Which expressions does the nurse use to cheer him up? ....

GRAMMAR

For/Since (depuis)

1. For

• Emploi

On emploie for pour parler d'une durée : for two seconds, for ten minutes, for two hours, for three days, for a week, for five months, for four years, for a long time, for ages, etc.

– This patient has been sleeping for two hours.

2. Since

• Emploi

On emploie since pour parler d'un point de départ : since two o'clock, since Christmas, since Saturday, since lunchtime, since 2001, since May, since he was twenty, since she arrived, etc.

– This patient has been sleeping since two o'clock.

• Remarque

Quand en français on utilise un présent, en anglais on utilise un present perfect ou un present perfect continuous en be + verbe en -ing.

– I've known him for thirteen years, since he was born, in fact: Je le connais depuis treize ans, en fait depuis qu'il est né.

– I have been working with him since this morning: Je travaille avec lui depuis ce matin.

Exercice 1

Réponse p. 104

Complétez par *since* ou *for*.

1. .... the end of last winter.
2. .... three years.
3. .... seven hours.
4. .... seven o'clock.
5. .... he broke his leg.
6. .... April.

Exercice 2

Réponse p. 104

Traduisez en anglais.

1. Depuis que je l'ai vu : ....
2. Depuis un quart d'heure : ....
3. Depuis le début de l'année : ....
4. Depuis son accident : ....
5. Depuis trois mois : ....

Exercice 3

Réponse p. 104

Mettez le verbe au bon temps, puis complétez par *since* ou *for*.

1. They (*know*) .... each other .... ten years.
2. He (*take*) .... this medication .... he was a child.
3. She (*be*) .... on a diet .... she left the clinic.
4. I (*not see*) .... her .... three days.
5. Mary (*be*) .... on duty .... Monday.

Travaillez à deux : How long...? (depuis combien de temps... ?)

Vous êtes deux infirmières. Posez les questions et répondez-y en utilisant les amorces suivantes.

Ex.: Work/in this unit.

A. How long have you been working in this unit?

B. I've been working in this unit since this morning.

1. know this surgeon.
2. be on the phone.
3. live in this country.
4. be ill.
5. be a nurse.
6. be married.

GRAMMAR

Adjectifs en -ed et en -ing

Un même radical peut avoir deux terminaisons différentes : -ed ou -ing.
Ex.: interested, interesting.

Ces deux adjectifs n'ont pas la même signification. Il ne faut pas les confondre.

Adjectif en -ed	Adjectif en -ing
Les adjectifs se terminant par -ed expriment une caractéristique ou un état d'une chose ou d'une personne. Ils correspondent, en français, aux adjectifs en -é.	Les adjectifs se terminant par -ing expriment une caractéristique ou un état qui agit sur les autres. Ils correspondent, en français, aux adjectifs en -ant.
I was interested in nursing when I was a child: Je m'intéressais au métier d'infirmière quand j'étais jeune.	I think nursing is a very interesting profession: Je pense que le métier d'infirmière est très intéressant.

Exercice 4

Réponse p. 104

Complétez les phrases avec les adjectifs suivants (au choix) :

1. He worked so much last night that he is .... today (*exhausting-exhausted*).
2. I'm not .... in this subject, even if it is .... (*interesting - interested*).
3. The way he speaks is .... (*shocked-shocking*)
4. It is................................, this is why I feel................................ (*embarrassed - embarrassing*).
5. He didn't succeed, his family was very................................ (*disappointing - disappointed*).

Travaillez à deux

En utilisant les adjectifs ci-dessus, posez des questions à votre partenaire commençant par *why*.

Ex.:

A. Why do you look so tired?

B. Because I went to bed late last night.

Exercice 5

Réponse p. 104

Donnez les contraires des adjectifs suivants.

Adjectifs	Contraires
rude	....
quiet	....
intolerant	....
shy	....
proud	....
boring	....
selfish	....
pessimistic	....

Piste 30

Exercice 6 : Intestinal problems

Traduction p. 212
Réponse p. 104

Écoutez le dialogue et complétez la conversation entre le médecin et sa patiente à l'aide des phrases suivantes :

- I take aspirin
- … … drink plenty of water to soften your faeces*
- … your stomach must be empty.
- but I didn't want to bother my family.
- … your bowels* using a fibreoptic tube.
- is there any blood in your stools*?

Patient You know, Doctor, I've always had intestinal problems, **(1)** ....

Doctor I see, well tell me, do you often take laxatives?

Patient Yes, because I'm often constipated.

Doctor But did you know they can actually disturb your digestive system?

Patient No, I didn't.

Doctor This is why you often have diarrhoea after taking the laxatives.

Patient And in addition, I have piles*, so when it's very painful **(2)** ....

Doctor And, tell me **(3)** .... ?

Patient No, there isn't.

Doctor Very well. As I mentioned, laxatives can disturb your digestive system, so you should eat a lot of fruit and **(4)** .... You'll have a colonoscopy tomorrow.

Patient Could you tell me what it is, please?

Doctor Yes, of course. We use a colonoscopy to check **(5)** ....
But before your intestinal examination **(6)** ....
So, first we'll give you a special liquid to drink to clear your bowels. It's nothing to worry about.

To help you

- **to soften your faeces:** ramollir vos selles
- **bowels:** intestins
- **stools:** selles
- **piles:** hémorroïdes

Piste 31 — Exercice 7

Réponse p. 104

Écoutez, puis répétez. Reliez chaque mot à son synonyme ou sa définition.

1. colonoscopy............ •
2. stools....................... •
3. gastroscopy............. •
4. roughage.................. •
5. examination............. •
6. piles......................... •

- • a. haemorrhoids
- • b. a bowel checkup
- • c. faeces
- • d. test
- • e. a stomach checkup
- • f. fibre

Piste 32 — Exercice 8 : Non Stéroidal Anti-Inflammatory Drugs (NSAIDs)

Réponse p. 104

Écoutez, puis répétez.

- stomach pain
- headache
- hives (urticaria)
- itching (pruritus)
- visual problems
- nausea
- vomiting
- reddening of the skin
- nervousness
- insomnia
- rash
- anxiety
- lack of appetite
- constipation
- diarrhea (US)/diarrhoea (GB)

Classez les effets indésirables des NSAIDs dans le tableau ci-dessous.

Side effects of Non Steroidal Anti-Inflammatory Drugs (NSAIDs)		
Digestive problems	**Central nervous problems**	**Skin problems**
....	....	....
....	....	....
....	....	....
....	....	....
....	....	....

Piste 33 — Exercice 9

Réponse p. 105

Après avoir lu les phrases ci-dessous, écoutez-les, puis complétez-les avec les prépositions que vous avez entendues.

1. My neighbour has been .... a diet for weeks.
2. She borrowed this bedpan .... the healthcare assistant.
3. The patient asked the doctor to call him .... as soon as he had the results.
4. You should give .... smoking. It's bad for your health.
5. The GP couldn't find .... what the disease was.
6. The paediatrician took the crying baby .... his arms.
7. He had never heard of this disease .... his studies.

Piste 34

Exercice 10

Réponse p. 105

Écoutez, puis répétez.

Complétez la légende avec les mots suivants :

- ureter
- kidney
- bladder
- urethra

Urinary system

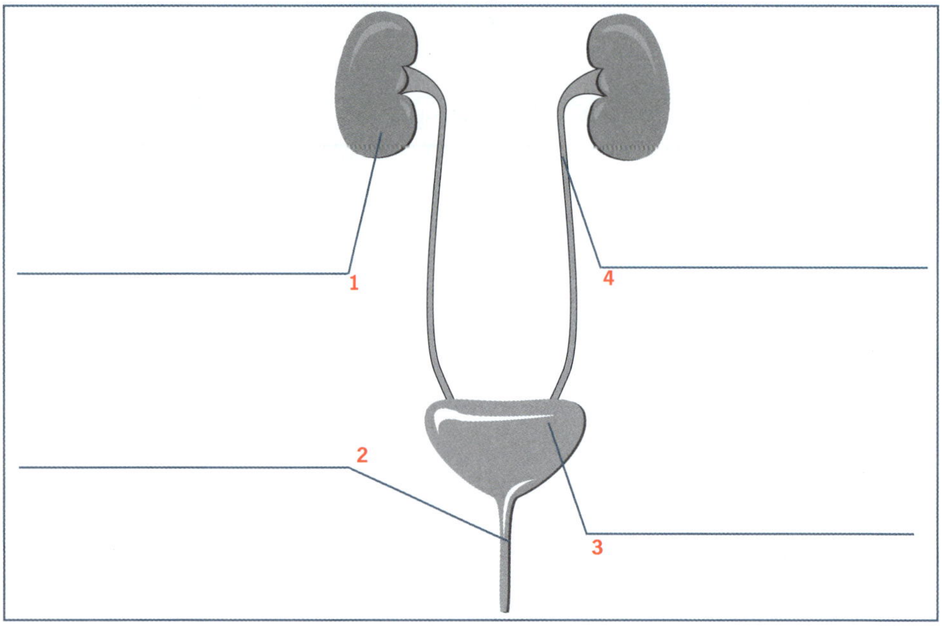

© C.K.

https://www.lienmini.fr/angsoin13

Travaillez à deux : Marginalization

"Marginalization leads to exclusion, oppression, discrimination and vulnerability."

Below is a list of people who experience marginalization. Choose one of these groups and explain to your partner how and why they become marginalized. Swap roles.

the poor
the uneducated
the elderly
the disabled
addicts (e.g. addicted to alcohol, drugs)
refugees
prostitutes
those with a psychiatric illness

Exercice 11 : Testez-vous !

Réponse p. 105

Traduisez en anglais.

1. Depuis quand avez-vous des problèmes intestinaux ? Depuis trois mois. En fait, depuis février.
....

2. De toute façon, elle n'a pas le moral depuis qu'elle est arrivée. ....
....

3. Ne vous inquiétez pas, tout va bien se passer. ....
....

4. Vous devez être à jeun avant cet examen. ....
....

5. Vous n'avez aucune raison d'avoir peur. ....
....

6. Cet anti-inflammatoire peut entraîner deux effets secondaires : des migraines et des douleurs d'estomac. ....
....

7. Elle a souvent des diarrhées après avoir pris des laxatifs. ....
....

Exercice 12 : Patient education

Réponse p. 105

Preventing infections in the hospital

Cochez la (les) bonne(s) affirmation(s).

	True	False
1. If you have diabetes, be sure that you and your doctor discuss the best way to control your blood sugar before, during, and after your hospital stay*. High blood sugar increases the risk of infection noticeably*.		
2. If you have an intravenous catheter, keep the skin around the dressing clean and dry.		
3. If you have a dressing on a wound, let your nurse know promptly if it works loose* or gets wet.		
4. Don't ask questions about your care so that you may fully understand your treatment plan.		
5. If you are overweight, losing weight will reduce the risk of infection following surgery.		

To help you

- **stay:** séjour
- **noticeably:** nettement
- **to work loose:** se défaire

https://www.lienmini.fr/angsoinq7a

Vocabulary quiz: Side effects

Réponse p. 105

Complétez chaque définition avec le terme correct.

1. A .... is an area of red spots on a person's skin, caused by an illness or an allergy.
a) nausea **b)** vomiting **c)** rash **d)** headache

2. The condition of being unable to get rid* of faeces* from the bowels is called ....
a) stomach pain **b)** constispation **c)** vomiting **d)** lack of appetite

3. A feeling of worry and anxiety is called ....
a) itching **b)** nervousness **c)** insomnia **d)** rash

4. You suffer from .... when you are unable to sleep.
a) urticaria **b)** diarrhea **c)** constipation **d)** insomnia

5. A .... is a continous pain in the head.
a) nervoussness **b)** headache **c)** itching **d)** stomach pain

https://www.lienmini.fr/angsoinq7bis

Vocabulary quiz

Réponse p. 105

Complétez chaque affirmation avec le terme correct.

1. You shouldn't drive because this medicine might make you feel ....
a) hot **b)** strong **c)** afraid **d)** dizzy*

2. You must stop using this drug immediately if your eyes are ....
a) cold **b)** itchy* **c)** allergic **d)** clean

3. You look pale and feel very weak*, so you must have ....
a) amnesia **b)** anaemia **c)** allergy **d)** anxiety

4. The GP gave me a .... for a new type of painkiller.
a) letter **b)** report **c)** prescription **d)** notice

5. The .... from this medication include stomach aches.
a) side effects **b)** stress **c)** asthma **d)** infection

To help you

- **to get rid of:** se débarrasser
- **faeces:** selles
- **to feel dizzy:** avoir des vertiges, des étourdissements
- **itchy:** qui pique(nt)
- **weak:** affaibli, faible

Medical Vocabulary: unit 7

- **faeces/stools:** selles
- **piles:** hémorroïdes
- **diarrhoea:** diarrhée
- **colonoscopy:** coloscopie
- **NIs:** infections nosocomiales
- **headache:** migraine
- **side effects:** effets secondaires
- **kidney:** rein
- **rash:** rougeur, plaque
- **bladder:** vessie
- **the elderly:** les personnes âgées

Let's discuss!

Population growth

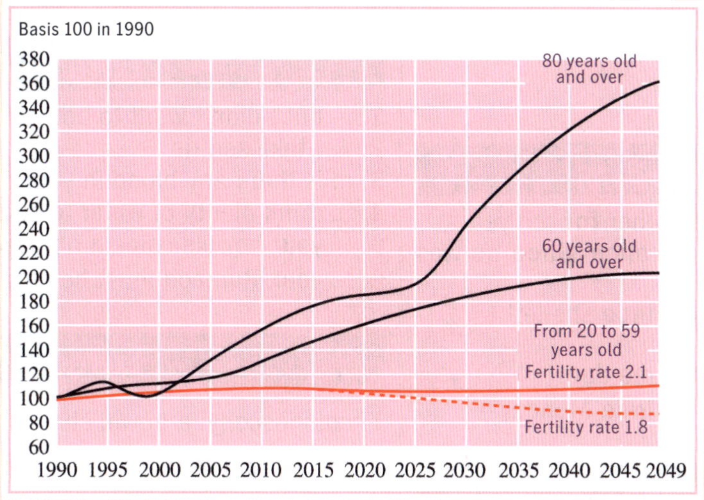

Comment on this graph.

How could you explain this population growth?

UNIT 7 Corrigés

Exercice 1

1. **Since** the end of last winter.
2. **For** three years.
3. **For** seven hours.
4. **Since** seven o'clock.
5. **Since** he broke his leg.
6. **Since** April.

Exercice 2

1. Since I saw him.
2. For a quarter of an hour.
3. Since the beginning of the year.
4. Since his/her accident.
5. For three months.

Exercice 3

1. They **have known** each other **for** ten years.
2. He **has taken** this medication **since** he was a child.
3. She **has been** on a diet **since** she left the clinic.
4. I **haven't seen** her **for** three days.
5. Mary **has been** on duty **since** Monday.

Exercice 4

1. exhausted 2. interested - interesting
3. shocking 4. embarrassing - embarrassed
5. disappointed.

Exercice 5

Adjectifs	Contraires
rude	polite
quiet	talkative
intolerant	tolerant
shy	sociable
proud	humble
boring	interesting
selfish	generous
pessimistic	optimistic

Exercice 6

1. ... but I didn't want to bother my family.
2. ... I take aspirin.
3. ... is there any blood in your stools?
4. ... drink plenty of water to soften your faeces.
5. ... your bowels using a fibreoptic tube.
6. ... your stomach must be empty.

Exercice 7

1. colonoscopy: a bowel checkup (b.)
2. stools: faeces (c.)
3. gastroscopy: a stomach checkup (e.)
4. roughage: fibre (f.)
5. examination: test (d.)
6. piles: haemorrhoids (a.)

Exercice 8

Side effects of Non Steroidal Anti-Inflammatory Drugs (NSAIDs)		
Digestive problems	**Central nervous problems**	**Skin problems**
stomach pain nausea vomiting diarrhoea constipation lack of appetite	headache visual problems insomnia, anxiety nervousness	hives (urticaria) itching (pruritus) reddening of the skin rash

Corrigés

Exercice 9

1. My neighbour has been **on** a diet for weeks.
2. She borrowed this bedpan **from** the healthcare assistant.
3. The patient asked the doctor to call him **back** as soon as he had the results.
4. You should give **up** smoking. It's bad for your health.
5. The GP couldn't find **out** what the disease was.
6. The paediatrician took the crying baby **in** his arms.
7. He had never heard of this disease **during** his studies.

Exercice 10

1. kidney 2. urethra 3. bladder 4. ureter

Exercice 11 : Testez-vous !

1. How long have you had intestinal problems? For three months. Since February, in fact.
2. She's been feeling down/depressed since she arrived.
3. Don't worry, everything will be all right.
4. Your stomach must be empty/you must have an empty stomach before this examination/test.
5. There is nothing to be afraid of.
6. This anti-inflammatory drug can lead to two side effects: headaches and stomach ache.
7. She often has diarrhoea after taking laxatives.

Exercice 12

1. True 2. True 3. True 4. False 5. True

Vocabulary quiz: Side effects

1. rash 2. constipation 3. nervousness 4. insomnia 5. headache

Vocabulary quiz

1. dizzy 2. itchy 3. anaemia 4. prescription 5. side effects

UNIT 8

UNIT 8

Giving advice and preventative care

Toutes les pistes audio de l'unité à télécharger ici
https://www.lienmini.fr/angsoinu8

Piste 35

Dialogue between Mr Brown and the nurse

Traduction pp. 212-213

Listen to the dialogue. A nurse is giving advice and preventative care to Mr Brown during his hospitalization.

Nurse We need to look at ways to prevent further complications for your heart and your diabetes.

Mr Brown OK, that sounds like a good idea.

Nurse Have you considered giving up smoking?

Mr Brown Yes, of course, but I'm afraid I won't be able to give up* by myself.

Nurse Well, I can suggest some support to help you.

Mr Brown Do you think it's possible to just give up instantly?

Nurse Yes, of course. You know some people take advantage of* their stay in hospital to give up and they succeed. Did you know your heart problem was due to tobacco?

Mr Brown No, I didn't.

Nurse And it's also due to the food you eat. You should think about going on a diet*.

Mr Brown Can you give me some advice on that?

Nurse Well, first of all, you are going to have to* cut down on* animal fats*, for example, cheese and butter. As part of your diet, you should also go easy on* meat that is high in fat, especially red meat.

Mr Brown Well, that's going to be difficult, I'm very keen on meat!

Nurse But you know, if you don't keep to your diet* you'll have problems. Sugar and sweets are also prohibited, but you are allowed to* use artificial sweeteners.

Mr Brown And, what about my weight?

Nurse Well, you do need to lose some weight. It would be a good idea to exercise regularly, walking, for example or cycling.

Mr Brown Well, thank you for your help. I'll do my best to follow your advice.

To help you

- **to give up:** arrêter de/cesser de
- **to take advantage of:** profiter de
- **to go on a diet:** suivre un régime
- **you are going to have to:** vous allez devoir
- **to cut down on:** réduire
- **fats:** graisses
- **to go easy on:** aller doucement
- **to keep to a diet:** bien suivre un régime
- **to be allowed to:** être autorisé/avoir le droit

Questions sur le dialogue

1. What does the nurse want to talk about and why? ....

....

2. What advice does she give about Mr Brown's diet? ....

....

3. What advice does she give about losing weight? ....

....

4. Do you think it'll be easy for Mr Brown to keep to this diet? Why or why not? ....

....

GRAMMAR

Modaux : exprimer l'obligation (must/to have to)

Attention, avec les modaux :
– pas de "s" à la 3e personne du singulier ;
– pas de "to" ni avant ni après ;
– les modaux servent d'auxiliaire dans les phrases négatives et interrogatives.

1. Must

• Emploi

Must exprime une obligation qui émane de soi, qui est personnelle.

• Construction

Forme affirmative	Sujet + must + verbe sans "to"	I must do it.
Forme négative	Sujet + must + not + verbe sans "to"	You must not forget your medicine.

• Remarque

Must ne s'emploie pas dans les formes interrogatives, on utilisera have to. Do I have to pay the doctor?
Conditionnel passé de must : He should have done it : Il aurait dû le faire.

2. To have to

• Emploi

Have to s'utilise lorsque l'obligation est extérieure : soit parce qu'une personne nous le demande, soit parce que les circonstances l'imposent.

• Construction

Forme affirmative	Sujet + have/has to + verbe	The patient has to go to the intensive care unit.
Forme négative	Sujet + don't/doesn't + have to + verbe	You don't have to leave now, visitors are allowed to stay from 4pm to 8pm.
Forme interrogative	Do/Does + sujet + have to + verbe	Does the patient have to take this tablet now?

• Remarque

"Do not (don't) have to" et "need not (needn't)" signifient : « Ce n'est pas obligé de ».
– You don't have to/needn't leave immediately: Vous n'êtes pas obligé de partir immédiatement.

8 UNIT

GRAMMAR

Modaux : donner un conseil (should)

• Emploi

Should et should not (shouldn't) servent à donner un conseil, un avis ou à exprimer une idée de devoir.

• Construction

Forme affirmative	Forme négative	Forme interrogative
Sujet + should + verbe	Sujet + should not (shouldn't) + verbe	(Mot interrogatif +) should + verbe
Children should eat a balanced diet.	You shouldn't judge patients.	What should I say to this patient?

• Remarque

On peut aussi utiliser must + verbe pour donner un conseil, le sens est alors plus fort et contient une idée de devoir : You must take your pills (sous-entendu, sinon vous aurez des problèmes de santé).

Exercice 1

Réponse p. 120

Complétez les phrases ci-dessous en utilisant *must, had to* ou *should.*

1. You .... smoke in the corridor, it's forbidden.
2. He .... be on a diet, because he was diabetic.
3. Children .... obey theirs parents, but some of them are very rude.
4. She .... follow my advice if she wants to get better.
5. The nurses were on strike, so the surgeon .... cancel two operations.

Piste 36

Exercice 2 : Nosocomial Infection (NI)

Réponse p. 120

Écoutez le texte une première fois ; puis complétez-le à la seconde écoute.

1. Patients who have long .... to multiple .... are at high .... of nosocomial infections.
2. The main aim of this unit is to .... nosocomial infections, through the identification of risk .... and to develop effective prevention measures.
3. To develop an infection .... hospitals should have an infection control ....
4. The .... of .... drips for blood transfusions can .... the risk of infection.

Piste 36

Exercice 3

Réponse p. 120

Écoutez. Puis cochez les cases : vrai ou faux ?

NIs have become a very serious problem in hospitals. To avoid germ transmission you must follow this advice.

	True	False
1. You must wash your hands frequently.	❑	❑
2. You mustn't use gloves to put up a drip.	❑	❑
3. You must use gloves to take a blood sample.	❑	❑
4. You must avoid germ transmission between one room and another.	❑	❑
5. You mustn't leave the dressing trolley* in the corridor.	❑	❑

To help you

- **dressing trolley:** chariot à pansements

Exercice 4 : Hand washing technique

Réponse p. 120

Réécrivez dans le bon ordre les instructions suivantes :

Before putting on gloves, a nurse must:

1. Throw the towel into the waste container.
2. Wipe hands with a sterile disposable towel.
3. Put on disposable gloves.
4. Wash and brush hands, wrists and forearms.

1. ....
2. ....
3. ....
4. ....

UNIT 8

Piste 37

Exercice 5 : In the cardiac care unit

Traduction p. 213
Réponse p. 120

Écouter le dialogue.
Puis complétez la conversation entre l'infirmier et le patient à l'aide des phrases suivantes :

- Please swallow it ...
- ... why I had a sharp pain in my chest
- ... to check your heart rate
- ... what is this device for?

Nurse You had a heart attack three days ago. The ECG[1] confirmed it. We had to do CPR[2]. So you'll have to stay in bed for a few days.

Patient Excuse me, can you tell me, is this the reason **(1)** .... and left arm?

Nurse Yes, that's right. I'll come and check your heart rate every two hours and do another ECG. Let's see your blood pressure now. Er... It's 140/80*. I'll just note it on your chart.

Patient And, sorry **(2)** ....

Nurse It records your heart rate, so I can see if everything is all right. I put two red dots* on your chest a few minutes ago **(3)** ....

Patient Is it possible to have another painkiller, please? I'm still in a lot of pain.

Nurse Certainly. Take this tablet. This should help you feel better. **(4)** .... don't let it dissolve*. All right?

Patient All right. Thanks.

Nurse You're welcome.

To help you

- **140/80:** se prononce one hundred and forty over eighty
- **a dot (here)/electrodes :** électrodes
- **to dissolve :** fondre

(1) *ECG (electrocardiogram).*
(2) *CPR (cardio pulmonary resuscitation).*

Exercice 6 : The heart

Réponse p. 120

Légendez le dessin du cœur avec les termes fournis ci-dessous.

- right auricle
- inferior veina cava
- pulmonary veina
- pulmonary artery
- aorta
- left auricle
- superior veina cava
- right ventricle
- left ventricle

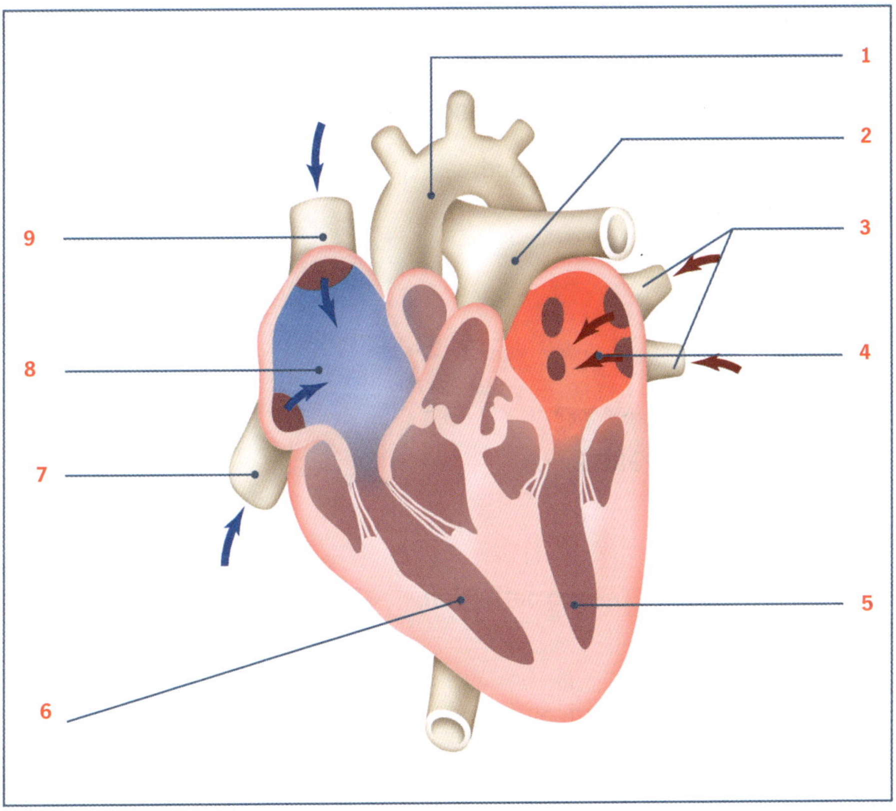

https://www.lienmini.fr/angsoin14

Piste 37 bis — Exercice 7 : Prononciation

Écoutez et répétez.

- a clot* in the lung: lung embolism
- a clot in the brain: brain embolism
- a clot in the leg: thrombosis

To help you

- **a clot:** un caillot

Exercice 8

Réponse p. 120

Écrivez en face de chaque définition le mot français correspondant.

1. Clot, semi-solid lump of coagulated blood: ....
2. Phlebitis, inflammation of the vein: ....
3. Cardiac arrest, heart failure: ....
4. Aneurysm: ....

Piste 38 — Exercice 9

Réponse p. 120

Écoutez, puis répétez.

Trouvez le mot qui correspond à chaque définition.

• lungs	• pharynx	• liver
• pancreas	• heart	• oesophagus

1. The gland near the stomach discharging a digestive secretion: ....
2. The tube leading from the mouth to the stomach: ....
3. The cavity behind the nose and mouth connecting them to the oesophagus: ....
4. The pair of organs used to draw air in and out: ....
5. The muscular organ maintaining the circulation of blood by contracting and dilating: ....
6. The glandular organ in the abdomen secreting bile: ....

Piste 39

Exercice 10

Réponse p. 121

Écoutez.

Puis complétez les fiches ci-dessous.

Salt-free diet	Low calorie diet	High fibre diet (for constipation)
In moderation	**Prohibited**	**In moderation**
Fish, liver, kidney	Oil, butter, margarine, milk	....
....	....	Cough medicine
Celery, spices	Sweets and alcoholic drinks	**Personal hygiene**
....	....	Go to the toilet at regular hours
Chocolate	Pulses*, meat high in fat	....
....	....	
Prohibited	**Advice**	**Allowed**
Pork, smoked ham	Do not nibble	....
....	....	Whole wheat bread
Seafood	Take artificial sweetener	....
....	....	Uncarbonated* beverages
Butter and margarine	Drink plenty of water	....
....	....	
Effervescent tablets		
....		

** Uncarbonated: non gazeux.*
** Pulses: légumes secs.*

Travaillez à deux : Advice on prevention

A: You are a patient and you ask advice on:

1. A low calorie diet.
2. A high fibre diet for constipation.
3. A salt-free diet.

B: You are a nurse. Give advice to this patient.

GRAMMAR

Adjectifs comparatifs

• Emploi

Les adjectifs au comparatif sont utilisés pour faire des comparaisons entre deux choses ou deux situations.

• Construction

Construction des phrases avec than :
– He illness is more serious than we thought.
– Doctors train longer than nurses.

1. Comparatifs de supériorité

Comparatifs réguliers	
Adjectifs courts (d'une syllabe ou deux) + -er + than	old ⇨ older than
Adjectif d'une syllabe finissant par -e + -r + than	safe ⇨ safer than
Adjectif de deux syllabes finissant par -y ⇨ -ier + than	easy ⇨ easier than
Adjectifs de deux syllabes ou plus + more + than	serious ⇨ more serious than

Comparatifs irréguliers
good/well ⇨ better (mieux, meilleur) far ⇨ farther/further (plus loin) bad ⇨ worse (pire, plus mauvais, plus mal)

2. Comparatifs d'égalité

On construit la phrase avec as + adjectif + as : His hands were as cold as ice.

3. Comparatifs d'infériorité

On construit les phrases en employant not as … as : An X-ray is not as good as a scan.

Exercice 11

Réponse p. 121

Complétez les phrases suivantes avec les adjectifs au comparatif en ajoutant *than* ou *as* quand c'est nécessaire.

• noisy	• painful	• good	• serious
• healthy	• near	• high	• tall

1. The nosocomial infection rate is .... in burns units .... in pediatric wards.
2. Her illness was .... we thought at first.
3. He couldn't sleep last night, he said: "This hospital is .... than a factory!"
4. Please, take this pain-killer, you'll feel ....
5. They are the same height: Paul is .... his sister.
6. I can't see the garden from here. I'd like to be a little .... the window.
7. You should eat more fruit. It's .... for you.
8. Her stomach ache is .... it was this morning.

Exercice 12 : Height and body weight

Réponse p. 121

Associez à chaque silhouette les adjectifs que vous utiliseriez pour décrire les caractéristiques par rapport à la taille, la minceur et la grosseur d'un patient.
Puis trouvez leurs équivalents français.

- large
- slim
- tall
- obese
- thin
- stout
- skinny
- average
- small/short
- overweight

Height

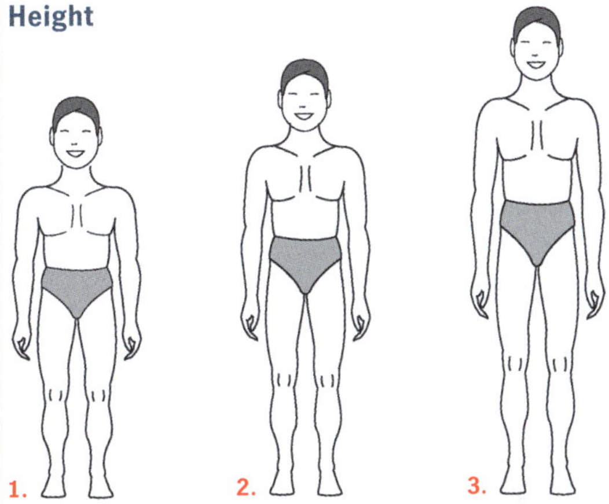

Body weight

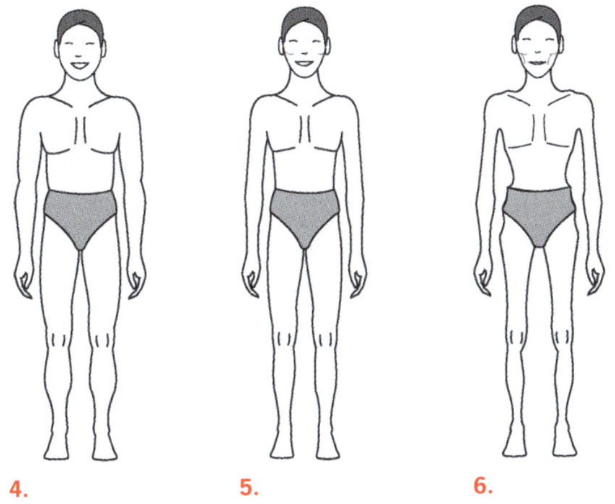

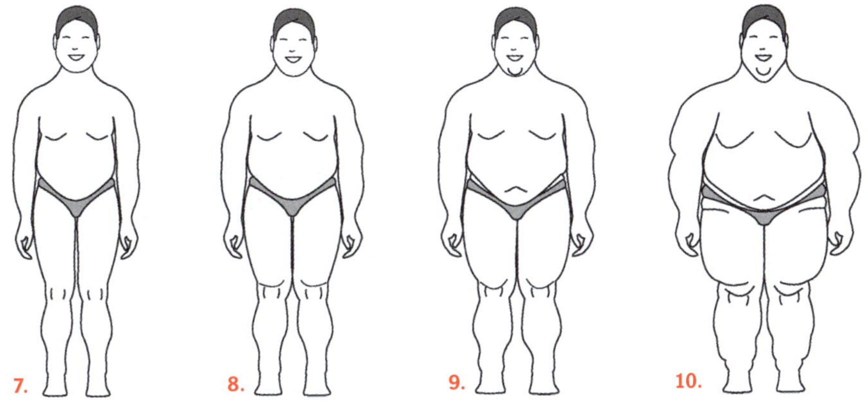

1. ....
2. ....
3. ....
4. ....
5. ....
6. ....
7. ....
8. ....
9. ....
10. ....

© C.K.

https://www.lienmini.fr/angsoin15

Exercice 13 : Testez-vous !

Réponse p. 122

Traduisez en anglais.

1. Il devait nous rappeler pour nous donner les résultats. ....

2. Vous devriez arrêter de fumer et bien suivre votre régime. ....

3. Je ne pourrai pas faire leurs pansements demain, je ne suis pas de service. ....

4. Pour éviter les infections nosocomiales, vous devriez laisser le chariot à pansement dans le couloir. ....

5. Le taux d'infection nosocomiale est moins élevé dans votre service que dans le nôtre. ....

6. À mon avis, travailler avec cette équipe est beaucoup plus intéressant. ....

Exercice 14 : Patient education

Réponse p. 122

How to reduce fat and cholesterol in your diet

Cochez la (les) bonne(s) affirmation(s).

	True	False
1. Eat fish or skinless* poultry* more often than beef or pork.		
2. Do not choose low-fat or non-fat dairy products* and cheese.		
3. Eat more grains, fresh fruit, vegetables, dried beans, and peas.		
4. Use vegetable fats instead of animal fats when cooking and limit the number of egg yolks* you eat to 2 or 3 per week.		
5. Do not limit meat portions.		

To help you

- **skinless:** sans la peau
- **poultry:** volaille
- **dairy product:** produit laitier
- **egg yolk:** jaune d'œuf

https://www.lienmini.fr/angsoinq8a

Verbs quiz: Diet

Réponse p. 122

Complétez chaque affirmation avec le verbe correct.

1. First of all, to .... a diet you have to cut down on cheese and butter.
a) give up **b)** go on **c)** lose **d)** go easy on

2. As part of his diet, he has to .... on red meat.
a) go easy **b)** have **c)** keep **d)** take advantage

3. He .... to eat animal fats once a week.
a) must **b)** can **c)** is allowed **d)** be able

4. You should .... on animals fats to go on a diet.
a) increase **b)** look for **c)** cut down **d)** eat

5. She can't .... smoking, she is a heavy smoker.
a) go on **b)** keep on **c)** start **d)** give up

https://www.lienmini.fr/angsoinq8b

Quiz on adjectives

Réponse p. 122

1. He is .... and has risk of heart disease, type 2 diabetes, high blood pressure, joint complications and certain cancers.
a) big **b)** tall **c)** obese **d)** average

2. They should eat more fruit, it is very .... for them.
a) serious **b)** healthy **c)** high **d)** easy

3. The doctor told her : « It is not ...., no need to worry. »
a) heavy **b)** simple **c)** serious **d)** strong

4. It was so .... he couldn't move his arm.
a) light **b)** tall **c)** painful **d)** skinny

5. An X-ray is not as .... as a scan.
a) better **b)** good **c)** best **d)** bad

Medical Vocabulary: unit 8

- **diet:** régime
- **ECG:** électrocardiogramme
- **clot:** caillot
- **BP/blood pressure:** tension artérielle
- **aneurysm:** anévrisme
- **overweight:** surpoids
- **lung:** poumon
- **dressing trolley:** chariot à pansement

Let's discuss!

Nosocomial infections

Nosocomial infections are contracted during hospitalization.

What are the different means of contamination? What are the consequences for the general public? What are the preventative measures?

Corrigés

Exercice 1

1. You **mustn't** smoke in the corridor, it's forbidden.
2. He **had to** be on a diet, because he was diabetic.
3. Children **should** obey theirs parents, but some of them are very rude.
4. She **must** follow my advice if she wants to get better.
5. The nurses were on strike, so the surgeon **had to** cancel two operations.

Exercice 2

1. Patients who have long **exposure** to multiple **antimicrobials** are at high **risk** of nosocomial infections.
2. The main aim of this unit is to **reduce** nosocomial infections, through the identification of risk **factors**. and to develop effective prevention measures.
3. To develop an infection **control programme** hospitals should have an infection control **committee**.
4. The **use** of **intravenous** drips for blood transfusions can **increase** the risk of infection.

Exercice 3

	True	False
1. You must wash your hands frequently.	✖	❑
2. You mustn't use gloves to put up a drip.	❑	✖
3. You must use gloves to take a blood sample.	✖	❑
4. You must avoid germ transmission between one room and another.	✖	❑
5. You mustn't leave the dressing trolley in the corridor.	❑	✖

Exercice 4

Before putting on gloves, a nurse must:

1. Wash and brush hands, wrists and forearms.
2. Wipe hands with a sterile disposable towel.
3. Throw the towel into the waste container.
4. Put on disposable gloves.

Exercice 5

1. why I had a sharp pain in my chest...
2. ... what is this device for?
3. ... to check your heart rate.
4. Please swallow it...

Exercice 6

1. aorta
2. pulmonary artery
3. pulmonary veina
4. left auricle
5. left ventricle
6. right ventricle
7. inferior veina cava
8. right auricle
9. superior veina cava

Exercice 8

1. clot, semi-solid lump of coagulated blood: caillot
2. phlebitis, inflammation of the vein: phlébite
3. cardiac arrest, heart failure: arrêt cardiaque
4. aneurysm: anévrisme

Exercice 9

1. pancreas
2. oesophagus
3. pharynx
4. lungs
5. heart
6. liver

Exercice 10

Salt-free diet	**Low calorie diet**	**High fibre diet** (for constipation)
In moderation	**Prohibited**	**In moderation**
Fish, liver, kidney	Oil, butter, margarine, milk	**Irritant laxatives**
Milk and cheese	**Pasta, rice, lentils**	Cough medicine
Celery, spices	Sweets and alcoholic drinks	
Instant coffee	**Sugar, honey, ice-cream**	**Personal hygiene**
Chocolate	Pulses, meat high in fat	Go to the toilet at regular hours
Biscuits	**Dried fruit**	**Physical exercise**
Prohibited	**Advice**	**Allowed**
Pork, smoked ham	Do not nibble	**Salads**
Pickled vegetables	**Eat three meals a day**	Whole wheat bread
	Take artificial sweetener	**Raw vegetables**
Seafood	**Reduce alcoholic beverages**	Uncarbonated beverages
Carbonated beverages		**Fruit, orange juice**
Butter and margarine	Drink plenty of water	
Salt	**Exercise regularly**	
Effervescent tablets		
Sodium bicarbonate		

Exercice 11

1. The nosocomial infection rate is **higher** in burns units **than** in paediatric wards.
2. Her illness was more **serious than** we thought at first.
3. He couldn't sleep last night, he said: "This hospital is **noisier** than a factory!"
4. Please, take this pain killer, you'll feel **better**.
5. They are the same height: Paul is **as tall as** his sister.
6. I can't see the garden from here. I'd like to be a little **nearer** the window.
7. You should eat more fruit. It's **healthier** for you.
8. Her stomach ache is **more painful** than it was this morning.

Exercice 12

1. small/short: petit
2. average: de taille moyenne
3. tall: grand
4. slim: mince
5. thin: maigre
6. skinny: squelettique
7. large: gros
8. stout: corpulent
9. overweight: en surcharge pondérale
10. obese: obèse

Corrigés

Exercice 13 : Testez-vous !

1. He had to call us back to give us the results.
2. You should stop/give up smoking and keep to your diet.
3. I won't be able to do their dressings tomorrow. I'm not on duty.
4. To avoid nosocomial infections you should leave your dressing trolley in the corridor.
5. The rate of nosocomial infection is lower on your ward than on ours.
6. In my opinion, working with this team is much more interesting.

Exercice 14

1. True
2. False
3. True
4. True
5. False

Verbs quiz: Diet

1. go on
2. go easy
3. is allowed
4. cut down
5. give up

Quiz on adjectives

1. obese
2. healthy
3. serious
4. painful
5. good

UNIT 9

UNIT 9

Preventing bedsores

Toutes les pistes audio de l'unité à télécharger ici
https://www.lienmini.fr/angsoinu9

Piste 40

Dialogue between Mr Brown and the nurse

Traduction p. 214

Listen to the dialogue. Mr Brown has been lying in bed for three weeks. His heels are painful. The nurse is explaining this is due to his long stay in bed. She is asking him questions to see whether there are any other complications.

Nurse Do you feel any other pain, stiffness* of the joints, for example?

Mr Brown No, only my heels hurt.

Nurse All right. Are you constipated at the moment?

Mr Brown No, I go to the toilet every morning.

Nurse Are you having difficulty breathing?

Mr Brown No. You know, I gave up smoking last Monday!

Nurse Congratulations. I've got a few more questions, if you don't mind. Does it hurt when you urinate?

Mr Brown No, not at all.

Nurse In order to prevent bedsores, you have to change your position from time to time. But if you need some help to do it tell us, a healthcare assistant will come and help you.

Mr Brown What about massages?

Nurse You'll have a massage once or twice a day. I'll put a cradle* on the bed to avoid having the weight of the blanket on your legs.

Mr Brown Well, that's nice of you. I was told* special mattresses, like water beds*, are used to prevent bedsores.

Nurse Yes, exactly. But yours is an air bed*. Don't forget you must drink lots of water to avoid getting dehydrated.

To help you

- **stiffness:** raideur
- **cradle:** arceau
- **I was told:** on m'a dit
- **water bed:** matelas à coussin d'eau
- **air bed:** matelas à coussin d'air

Questions sur le dialogue

1. How long has Mr Brown been in bed? ....

....

....

2. What does he have to do to prevent bedsores? ....

....

....

3. List the different mattresses used to prevent bedsores. ....

....

....

4. What other advice would you give to a patient to prevent bedsores? ....

....

....

GRAMMAR

Modaux : exprimer la possibilité et la capacité (can / could / may / might)

• Sens

1. Can/could

Ils expriment :

– une possibilité liée au présent pour can et liée au passé pour could ;

– une capacité : I can speak English.

Remarque :
Au futur, la capacité se traduit par be able to : I will be able to come.
Conditionnel passé de can: He could have done it: Il aurait pu le faire.

2. May/might

Ils expriment également une possibilité mais aussi l'éventualité de situations à venir.

3. Might

Il exprime une possibilité, un risque, une suggestion.

• Construction

Forme affirmative	Sujet + can/could/may/might + infinitif sans "to"	You could work in this hospital next year.
Forme négative	Sujet + may/might + not + infinitif sans "to"	This patient might not be able to leave tomorrow.
Forme interrogative	Might/Could + sujet + infinitif sans "to"	Could she loose consciousness?
	Mot interrogatif + might/could + sujet + infinitif sans "to"	What advice could you give him?

Exercice 1

Réponse p. 136

Complétez les phrases ci-dessous avec les modaux suivants :

• might	• could	• shouldn't	• may
• must	• won't have to	• needn't	

1. You .... drink so much. It's bad for your health.
2. She .... have an X-ray tomorrow.
3. .... you please come and fetch me from hospital at 4 p.m.?
4. You .... take this medicine tonight.
5. .... I borrow your stethoscope, please?
6. You .... sit in the waiting room before seeing the doctor.
7. She .... come with her husband, but it isn't certain.

Exercice 2

Réponse p. 136

Complétez les phrases ci-dessous en utilisant *can* ou *could*.

1. We .... see more and more people dying of AIDS in developing countries.
2. She asked me if I .... answer the phone because she was very busy.
3. If you don't have enough time you .... tell me.
4. If only he .... stop smoking!
5. I told him, he .... let me know if he had the information.

Travaillez à deux : Asking for permission

A asks for permission: May I ....?
B refuses and gives a reason.

A wants to:

1. have a painkiller. ....
2. drink some water. ....
3. talk to the cardiologist. ....
4. have a shower. ....
5. have my drip removed. ....
6. walk to the visitor's room. ....

Exercice 3

Réponse p. 136

Associez un élément de chaque colonne afin de composer des phrases cohérentes.

1. I couldn't fill in the forms....... •
2. She must stay in bed.............. •
3. You needn't.............................. •
4. You should not take.................. •
5. I don't know who...................... •

- .... **A.** come tomorrow.
- .... **B.** so many pills.
- .... **C.** because I was in a hurry.
- .... **D.** for a couple of days.
- .... **E.** is on duty next week-end.

Piste 41

Exercice 4

Réponse p. 136

Écoutez les phrases suivantes : qui parle ? L'infirmier, le médecin ou le patient ?

	Nurse	Doctor	Patient
1. I have to examine you. You are suffering from chest pains.	❑	❑	❑
2. I have to give him his medication at 10:30.	❑	❑	❑
3. I don't have to give him an injection right now.	❑	❑	❑
4. I often have to explain to a convalescent that he needs sleep.	❑	❑	❑
5. I have to go to the physiotherapist once a week.	❑	❑	❑
6. It's great, I don't have to have any more blood transfusions.	❑	❑	❑

Travaillez à deux

Reprenez les phrases de l'exercice 4 puis posez à votre partenaire des questions en vous en inspirant.

A. Why do you have to examine me?

B. I have to examine you because you are suffering from chest pains.

....

....

....

....

....

....

....

....

Exercice 5 : Preventing bedsores

Réponse p. 136

Complétez les légendes des différentes localisations des escarres à l'aide des mots placés sous chaque dessin.

Dorsal decubitus

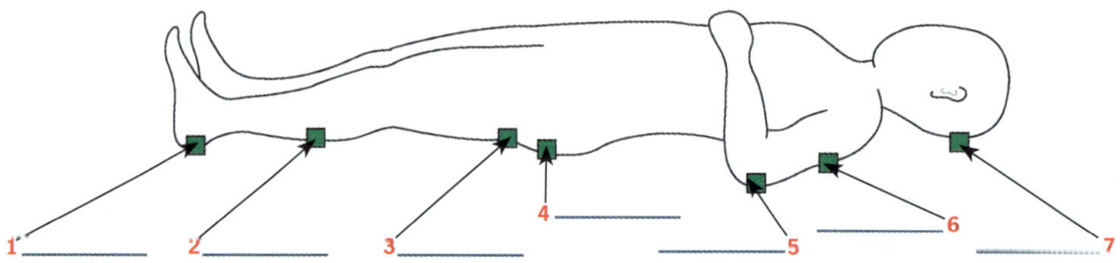

skull	ischium	heel	elbow	scapula	sacrum	calf

Left or right decubitus

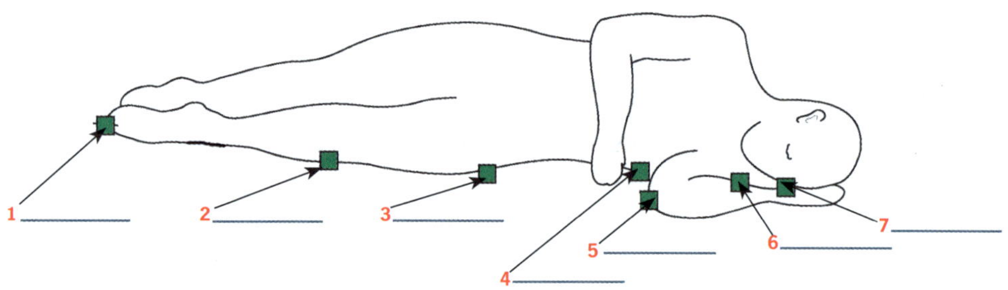

knee	foot	rib	elbow	hip	ear	shoulder

Ventral decubitus

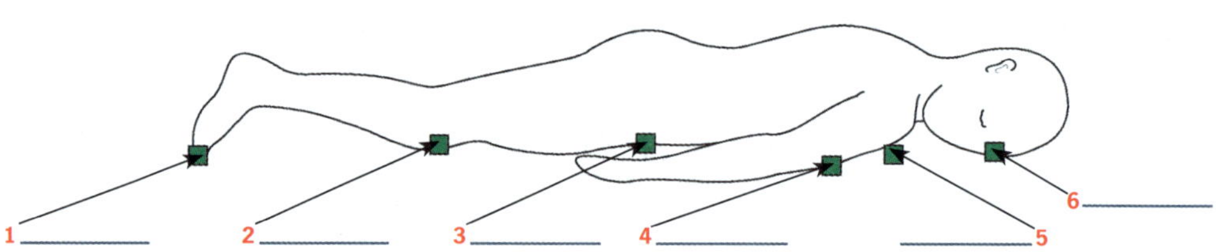

toes	male genitals	shoulder	cheek and ear	knee	breasts

https://www.lienmini.fr/angsoin16

Piste 42

Exercice 6 : Giving pre-medication

Traduction p. 214
Réponse p. 136

Écoutez le dialogue.

Puis complétez la conversation entre l'infirmier et la patiente à l'aide des phrases suivantes :

- A little anxious, I must admit
- ... under observation
- Can you stretch out your arm, please

In the surgical ward.

Nurse Good morning Mrs White. You are going for your operation in a while. I'm just going to give you a little injection. It will help you to relax a little before your operation **(1)** .... How do you feel?

Patient **(2)** ....

Nurse Don't worry, everything will be all right. We'll tell your husband when the operation is over.

Patient Has he given you the consent form*?

Nurse Yes, he has.

After the operation, in the recovery room*.

Nurse Mrs White, the operation went smoothly*, but we'll keep you **(3)** .... for a while. I'm just going to give you some oxygen. I know it isn't very pleasant but try to relax. Breathe normally, please. That's it. Take it easy. You'll see your husband in a moment.

To help you

- **consent form:** autorisation d'opérer
- **recovery room:** salle de réveil
- **to go smoothly:** s'être bien passé

UNIT 9

GRAMMAR

Adjectifs superlatifs

• Emploi

Les adjectifs superlatifs sont utilisés pour faire des comparaisons entre plus de deux choses ou situations.

• Construction

Superlatifs réguliers	
Adjectifs courts (d'une syllabe ou deux) + the -est	old ⇨ the oldest
Adjectif de deux syllabes finissant par -y + the -y ⇨ -iest	greedy ⇨ the greediest
Adjectifs de deux syllabes ou plus + the most	Serious ⇨ the most serious

Superlatifs irréguliers
good/well ⇨ the best (le mieux, le meilleur) bad/badly ⇨ the worst (le pire, le plus mauvais) far ⇨ the farthest/the furthest (le plus loin, le plus éloigné) less ⇨ the least (le moins)

• Exemples

This is the safest medication we have.
She has the most serious type of fracture.
This is the best medication for your illness.

• Remarques

Il faut distinguer most et most of.
Most traduit : la plupart, la majorité, la plus grande partie de. Il exprime une généralité : Most patients are afraid of pain.
Most of est employé devant un déterminant (ex.: the, this) ou un pronom (ex.: us, them) : Most of the patients I know are afraid of pain.

Exercice 7

Réponse p. 137

Complétez les phrases avec les adjectifs suivants au superlatif.

• expensive • bad • frequent • high • low

1. Magnetic Resonance Imaging (MRI) is one of .... imaging techniques.
2. .... percentage of obese people can currently be found in the USA.
3. Respiratory diseases are .... cause of death during the perinatal period.
4. It's in our paediatric department that the infection rate is ....
5. .... experience he had was his car accident last week.

Piste 43 — Travaillez à deux

Écoutez les phrases.
Dites chacun votre tour si vous êtes ou non d'accord avec ces affirmations : *I agree/disagree with this statement because…*

1. Doctors should give patients all the information necessary about their condition.
2. Kidney transplants should be stopped, because they are seldom successful.
3. People who suffer a lot should have the right to decide whether they want to terminate their lives.
4. The tax on alcohol should be increased.
5. Therapeutic cloning should be stopped.

Exercice 8

Réponse p. 137

Associez un élément de chaque colonne afin de composer des phrases cohérentes.

Many factors increase the risk of nosocomial infections .... •	• .... because some are absorbed by the liver.
He exercises too vigorously........................ •	• .... whereas few affect the risk of specific infection.
Backache and torn muscles could be avoided .... •	• .... in order to prevent disease spreading.
Vaccination programmes are used............ •	• .... consequently he sprained his calf muscle last week.
Hormone tablets are less effective when taken orally.. •	• .... on condition a little care is taken.

Piste 44 — Exercice 9

Réponse p. 137

Écoutez, puis complétez les phrases suivantes avec un mot de liaison.

1. .... she doesn't take this capsule, she won't get better.
2. They got sunburn .... they had put on suntan lotion.
3. He is still convalescing, ... his sister has already recovered.
4. .... he is unable to make up his mind, I made the decision for him.
5. Drug-addiction is getting more and more prevalent ....in poor nations.
6. You'll have to wait .... Doctor Burns comes back.
7. He is very weak .... the blood transfusion.

Quels sont leurs équivalents français ?

1. ....
2. ....
3. ....
4. ....
5. ....
6. ....
7. ....

Piste 45

Exercice 10

Réponse p. 137

Écoutez, puis répétez.

Complétez la légende à l'aide des mots suivants :

- lung
- windpipe/trachea
- nose
- bronchi
- diaphragm

Respiratory system

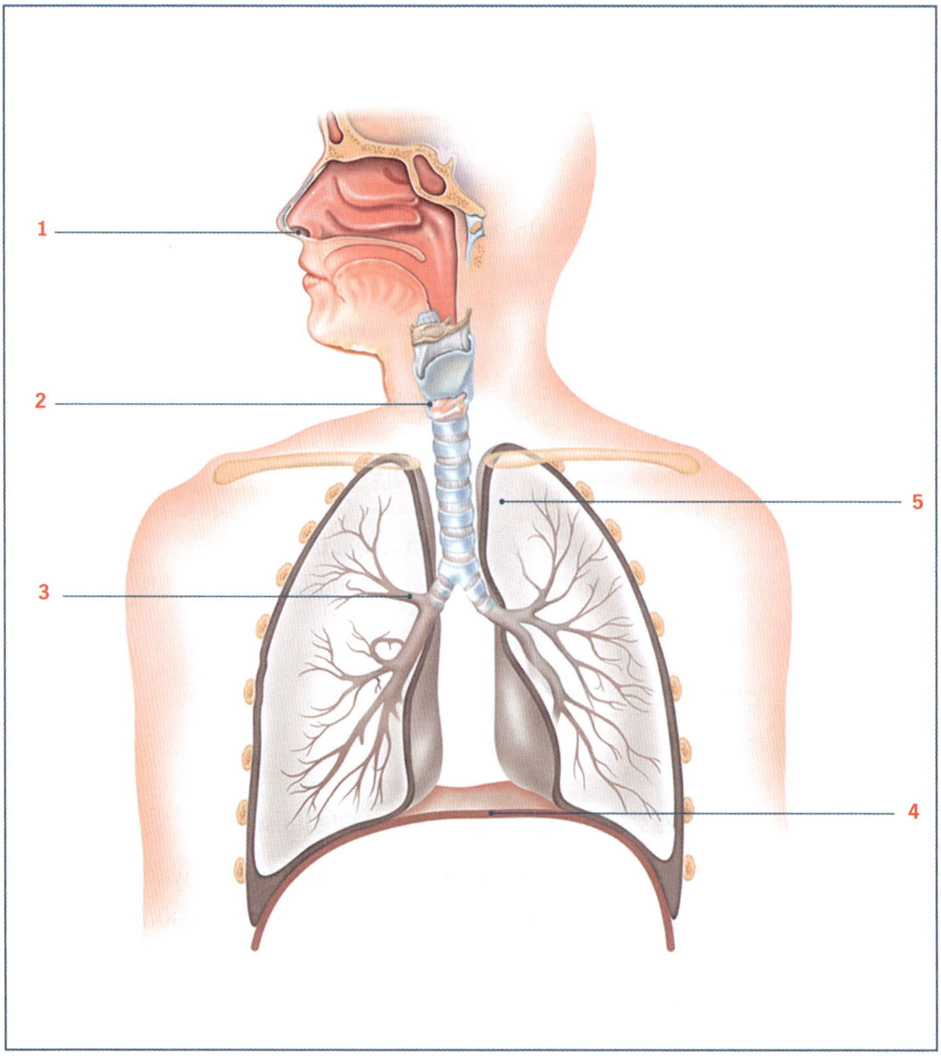

https://www.lienmini.fr/angsoin17

Exercice 11 : Testez-vous !

Réponse p. 137

Traduisez en anglais.

1. Il se peut que l'IRM soit l'un des systèmes d'imagerie les plus cher. ....

2. Vous n'êtes pas obligé de lui dire qu'ils sont rarement à l'heure. ....

3. Elle s'est foulée la cheville hier. Par conséquent, elle ne pourra pas venir avec nous demain. ..

4. Tu n'es jamais d'accord avec eux, ce que je regrette sincèrement. ....

5. Il se pourrait qu'ils le mettent sous oxygène pendant un moment. ....

6. Selon lui, le traitement hormonal était le moins efficace. ....

7. Bien qu'elle prenne ce traitement depuis des mois, elle ne se sent pas mieux. ....

Exercice 12 : Patient education

Réponse p. 137

Medication adherence*

Cochez la (les) bonne(s) affirmation(s).

	True	False
1. Patients never test the effect of stopping the medicine or altering the dosage in relation to their symptoms.		
2. Adherence programs have focused on simplifying dosage and delivery, patient education and modifying patient behaviour.		
3. There are different ways to remind patients to take medication : pill organizers, calendars and phone reminder systems.		
4. It is not important for the patient to visit the pharmacy to discuss adherence.		
5. It is essential to understand the reasons why the patient may not want or is unable to take his/her treatment.		

To help you

- **medication adherence:** adhésion au traitement/observance du traitement

https://www.lienmini.fr/angsoinq9a

Verbs quiz

Réponse p. 138

Complétez chaque affirmation avec le verbe correct.

1. The surgeon .... last night.
a) made b) operated c) did d) called

2. The physician .... me a prescriptions for antibiotics.
a) gave b) made c) read d) did

3. A catheter is a thin tube that is.. the body to remove urine.
a. made b. used c. put into d. taken

4. The nurses .... the children until their parent's return.
a. look at b. look for c. look after d. look through

5. I don't .... very well, I'm sick.
a) fall b) felt c) feel d) fell

http://www.lienmini.fr/angsoinq9b

Vocabulary quiz

Réponse p. 138

Complétez chaque affirmation avec le terme correct.

1. Backache could be avoided on condition little .... is taken.
a) pain b) care c) time d) techniques

2. The Magnetic Resonance Imaging (MRI) might be one of the most .... imaging technique.
a) cheap b) long c) expensive d) oldest

3. Hormone tablets are less .... when taken orally.
a) efficient* b) serious c) effective* d) frequent

4. Vaccination programmes are used in order to prevent disease ....
a) reduction b) spreading c) decreasing d) cutting

5. The .... percentage of obese people can currently be found in the USA.
a) lowest b) best c) worse d) highest

To help you

- **efficient:** efficace (pour une personne)
- **effective:** efficace (pour une chose)

Medical Vocabulary: unit 9

- **bedsore:** escarre
- **consent form:** autorisation d'opérer
- **MRI:** IRM
- **physiotherapist:** kinésithérapeute
- **intensive care unit (ICU):** unité de soins intensifs
- **surgical ward:** chirurgie
- **backache:** lombalgie
- **torn muscle:** déchirure musculaire
- **windpipe:** trachée

Let's discuss!

Nurse: a difficult occupation.

- "At the end of the day, I have the pleasure of knowing that my job is useful; that I've done something really important". Sandrine L.
- "Certainly there are numerous disadvantages: a schedule that conflicts with family life, insufficient salary compared to the level of responsibility, physical and mental exhaustion*. But it's a job that I love with all its 'ups and downs', even if we don't have enough time to do it as well as we would like." Denis B.

Discuss the advantages and disadvantages of nursing presented in these two points of view.

To help you

- **exhaustion:** grande fatigue

9 UNIT

Corrigés

Exercice 1

1. You **shouldn't** drink so much. It's bad for your health.
2. She **won't** have to have an X-ray tomorrow.
3. **Could** you please come and fetch me from hospital at 4 p.m.?
4. You **needn't** take this medicine tonight.
5. **May** I borrow your stethoscope, please?
6. You **must** sit in the waiting room before seeing the doctor.
7. She **might** come with her husband, but it isn't certain.

Exercice 2

1. We **can** see more and more people dying of AIDS in developing countries.
2. She asked me if I **could** answer the phone because she was very busy.
3. If you don't have enough time you **can** tell me.
4. If only he **could** stop smoking!
5. I told him, he **could** let me know if he had the information.

Exercice 3

1. I couldn't fill in the forms……	→ C	**A.** come tomorrow.
2. She must stay in bed……………	→ D	**B.** so many pills.
3. You needn't…………………………	→ A	**C.** because I was in a hurry.
4. You should not take………………	→ B	**D.** for a couple of days.
5. I don't know who…………………	→ E	**E.** is on duty next week-end.

Exercice 4

	Nurse	Doctor	Patient
1. I have to examine you. You are suffering from chest pains.	❑	✖	❑
2. I have to give him his medication at 10:30.	✖	❑	❑
3. I don't have to give him an injection right now.	✖	✖	❑
4. I often have to explain to a convalescent that he needs sleep.	✖	✖	❑
5. I have to go to the physiotherapist once a week.	❑	❑	✖
6. It's great, I don't have to have any more blood transfusions.	❑	❑	✖

Exercice 5

Dorsal decubitus: 1. heel; 2. calf; 3. ischium; 4. sacrum; 5. elbow; 6. scapula; 7. skull.

Left or right decubitus: 1. foot; 2. knee; 3. hip; 4. rib; 5. elbow; 6. shoulder; 7. ear.

Ventral decubitus: 1. toes; 2. knee; 3. male genitals; 4. breasts; 5. shoulder; 6. cheek and ear.

Exercice 6

1. Can you stretch out your arm, please?
2. A little anxious, I must admit.
3. ... under observation.

Exercice 7

1. Magnetic Resonance Imaging (MRI) is one of **the most expensive** imaging techniques.
2. **The highest** percentage of obese people can currently be found in the USA.
3. Respiratory diseases are **the most frequent** cause of death during the perinatal period.
4. It's in our paediatric department that the infection rate is **the lowest**.
5. **The worst** experience he had was his car accident last week.

Exercice 8

- Many factors increase the risk of nosocomial infections .... whereas few affect the risk of specific infection.
- He exercises too vigorously .... consequently he sprained his calf muscle last week.
- Backache and torn muscles could be avoided .... on condition a little care is taken.
- Vaccination programmes are used .... in order to prevent disease spreading.
- Hormone tablets are less effective when taken orally .... because some are absorbed by the liver.

Exercice 9

1. **If (si)** she doesn't take this capsule, she won't get better.
2. They got sunburn **although (bien que)** they had put on suntan lotion.
3. He is still convalescing, **while (alors que)** his sister has already recovered.
4. **Since (puisque)** he is unable to make up his mind, I made the decision for him.
5. Drug-addiction is getting more and more prevalent **even (même)** in poor nations.
6. You'll have to wait **until (jusqu'à ce que)** Doctor Burns comes back.
7. He is very weak **in spite of (malgré)** the blood transfusion.

Exercice 10

1. nose
2. windpipe/trachea
3. bronchi
4. diaphragm
5. lung

Exercice 11 : Testez-vous !

1. The Magnetic Resonance Imaging (MRI) may be one of the most expensive imaging techniques.
2. You don't have to/needn't tell him/her they are rarely on time.
3. She sprained her ankle yesterday. Consequently she won't be able to come with us tomorrow.
4. You never agree with them, which I sincerely regret.
5. They might put him under oxygen for a while.
6. According to him, the hormone treatment was the least effective.
7. Even though she was taking this treatment for months, she doesn't feel better.

Exercice 12

1. False
2. True
3. True
4. False
5. True

Corrigés

Verbs quiz

1. operated
2. gave
3. put into
4. look after
5. feel

Vocabulary quiz

1. care
2. expensive
3. effective
4. spreading
5. highest

UNIT 10

UNIT 10

Dealing with conflict*

Toutes les pistes audio de l'unité à télécharger ici
https://www.lienmini.fr/angsoinu10

Piste 46

Dialogue between Mr Neil and the nurse

Traduction p. 215

Listen to the dialogue. Mr Neil, one of Mr Brown's close friends, has come to visit him. He's coming out of Mr Brown's room and seems very angry.

Mr Neil I've just spoken to my friend and his back is very painful. Can't you do something to help with the pain?

Nurse We're doing our best, but Mr Brown is a little reserved, he doesn't tell us when he is in pain.

Mr Neil It doesn't matter*! He's been here for three weeks now and I think you could have done something to relieve the pain, don't you think?

Nurse Unfortunately, Mr Brown had some complications as well, which didn't make things any easier.

Mr Neil Right, and I'd like to get information about these complications. It's impossible to get any information in this hospital!

Nurse Unfortunately, I can't tell you anything about it, I'm afraid. It's a question of patient confidentiality*. However, I'd like to take advantage of your visit to ask you some questions about Mr Brown. You may have information about him that could be helpful for us. Is that possible?

Mr Neil Sure, no problem.

Nurse Would you like a cup of coffee?

Mr Neil Yes, OK.

To help you

- **to deal with conflict:** faire face à un conflit
- **it doesn't matter:** ça ne fait rien
- **by the way:** à propos
- **patient confidentiality:** secret professionnel

Questions sur le dialogue

1. Why is Mr Neil angry? ....
....
2. Do you think Mr Neil was right to speak to the nurse in this way? Why or why not? ....
....
3. Why is it so hard to estimate the degree of pain? ....
....
4. Is patient confidentiality necessary? Why or why not? ....
....
5. How would you have dealt with such a situation? ....
....

GRAMMAR

Conditionnel

1. Conditionnel présent

• Emploi

Le conditionnel permet de parler de choses qui ne sont pas sûres :

- If I knew Mr Neil's number I would phone him: Si je connaissais le numéro de M. Neil je lui téléphonerai.

Il s'emploie comme le conditionnel français avec la conjonction if :

- The procedure would be easier if he had the right scalpel: La procédure serait plus facile s'il avait le bon scalpel.

• Construction

Forme affirmative	Forme négative	Forme interrogative
Sujet + would + infinitif sans "to"	Sujet + would not (wouldn't) + infinitif sans "to"	Would + sujet + infinitif sans "to"
I would (I'd) do it if I had the time.	If they had the choice they wouldn't perform the operation.	What would you do if you had lung cancer?

• Remarque

Pas de conditionnel après when, as soon as, while mais un prétérit : She said she would call me when she arrived.

2. Conditionnel passé

Construction : would have + participe passé

- He would have written the report if he had received the results: Il aurait écrit le rapport s'il avait reçu les résultats.

UNIT 10

Exercice 1

Réponse p. 152

Complétez les phrases suivantes en utilisant le temps correct.

1. If I knew her name I .... you. (*introduce*)
2. If he had arrived earlier you .... him. (*meet*)
3. He told her he would type the letter as soon as he .... the information. (*have*)
4. I .... on you if it was possible. (*operate*)
5. If you had arrived on time I .... it this morning. (*can do*)

Exercice 2

Réponse p. 152

Mettez les verbes suivants à la forme correcte.

1. I would travel if I.. enough timex (*have*).
2. If I see Denis I .... him the medical report (*give*).
3. If I had known I .... them (*invite*).
4. If he (*know*) .... what was going to happen, he (*do*) .... something about it.
5. We .... his treatment if he feels better (*stop*).

Travaillez à deux

Posez à votre partenaire les questions suivantes en commençant par : *What would you do if...* Puis inversez les rôles.

1. A patient woke you up in the middle of the night?
2. You were the first to arrive at the scene of a car accident?
3. Your child had a minor burn?
4. A patient had swallowed some kind of poison?
5. A patient was crying?

Exercice 3

Réponse p. 152

Entourez l'intrus de chaque liste.

1. **Diseases**	:	tetanus	–	diphtheria	–	breast	–	yellow fever
2. **Parts of the head**	:	nose	–	ear	–	hip	–	forehead
3. **Joints**	:	elbow	–	ankle	–	cheek	–	neck
4. **Eye**	:	eyelid	–	flu	–	iris	–	lens
5. **Bones**	:	skull	–	cornea	–	rib	–	spine
6. **Organs**	:	spleen	–	toe	–	bladder	–	heart

Piste 47

Exercice 4 : Childhood diseases

Réponse p. 152

Écoutez, puis répétez.

- whooping cough
- meningitis
- ear infection
- measles
- chickenpox
- polio
- rubella/German measles
- mumps
- diphtheria

Complétez la liste des maladies ci-dessous avec leur traduction en anglais :

1. diphtérie : ....
2. rougeole : ....
3. rubéole : ....
4. méningite : ....
5. varicelle : ....
6. oreillons : ....
7. otite : ....
8. poliomyélite : ....
9. coqueluche : ....

Travailler à deux

Que diriez-vous à ces personnes dans les situations suivantes ?

Posez la question à votre voisin puis échangez les rôles : "*What would you say if…?/What would you do if…?*"

1. .... if one of your friends was a heavy drinker.
2. .... if your sister only saw a gynaecologist very occasionally.
3. .... if your child was overweight.
4. .... if your colleague smoked a packet of cigarettes a day.
5. .... if your mother didn't have a check-up every year.

Piste 48

Exercice 5

Réponse p. 152

Écoutez, puis répétez.

Complétez la légende à l'aide des mots suivants :

- potty
- bottle
- incubator
- nappy
- teddy bear
- dummy
- teat
- comfort blanket

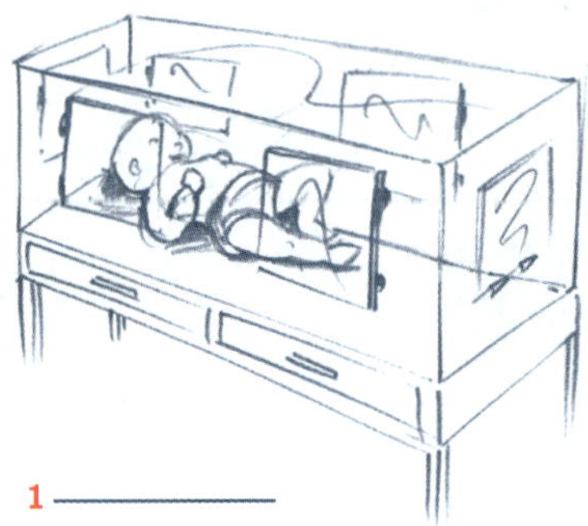

1 ____________

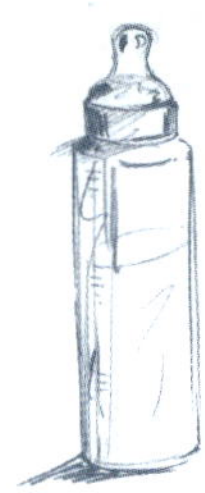

2 ____________

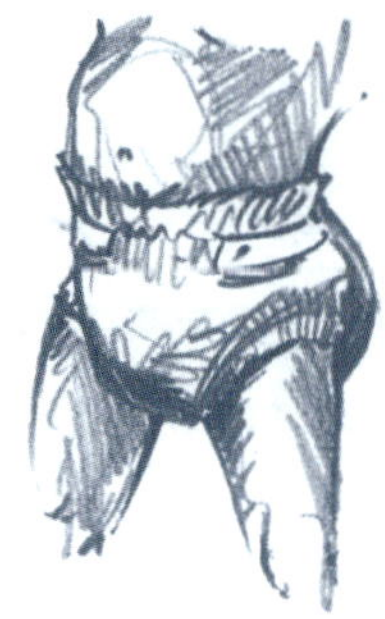

3 ____________

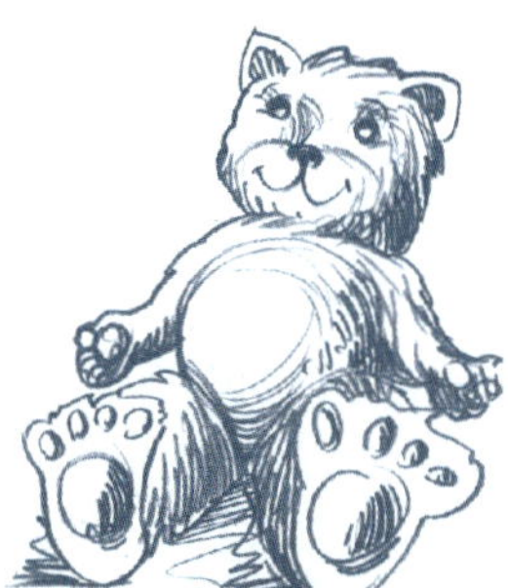

4 ____________

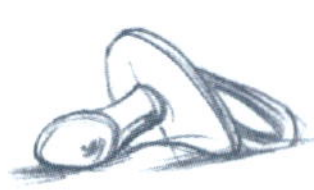

5 ____________

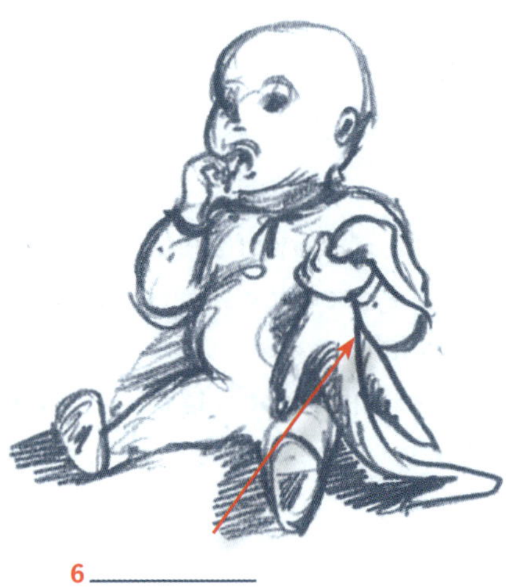

6 ____________

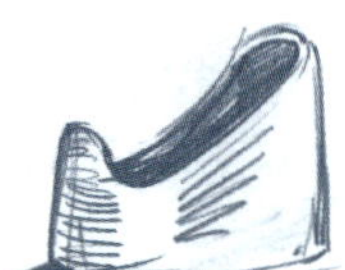

7 ____________

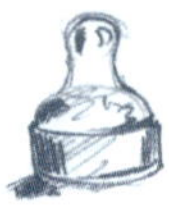

8 ____________

https://www.lienmini.fr/angsoin18

Exercice 6 : The paediatric ward

Piste 49

Traduction p. 215
Réponse p. 152

Écoutez le dialogue et complétez la conversation entre l'infirmière et la mère d'un bébé. Utilisez les phrases suivantes :

- I'll change your nappy...
- ... he keeps on scratching his left ear.
- What's his sleeping pattern like?
- ... is fond of his comfort-blanket.
- ... all his vaccinations*?
- ... we have to keep your little baby in...

Talking to the mother.

Nurse I'm sorry but **(1)** .... for a few days.

Mother Why?

Nurse Well, he's got a high temperature because of his ear infection.

Mother This is why **(2)** ....

Nurse Yes exactly. Tell me, are you up to date with* **(3)** ....

Mother Yes, I am.

Nurse And does he usually sleep with a dummy?

Mother No, but Brian **(4)** .... I've brought it with me. Here it is.

Nurse Thank you. **(5)** ....

Mother He needs a nap* in the afternoon. Can I stay to nurse* him?

Nurse Well of course and it'll be much better for him.

Talking to the baby.

Nurse Your mummy and daddy are going home now. They need some rest, but don't worry they'll come back tomorrow and I'll be here with you tonight. **(6)** ...., it's all wet. All right? Night night* Brian...

10 UNIT

To help you

- **vaccination** = vaccin
- **to be up to date with:** être à jour de
- **nap:** sieste
- **to nurse/to breast feed:** allaiter
- **night night:** bonne nuit (à un enfant)

Travaillez à deux : Pain in children

How do children communicate pain?

Face scales can often be used with children. They can communicate their pain by pointing to one of the faces.

Use the face scale below and practice asking a child about his or her pain.

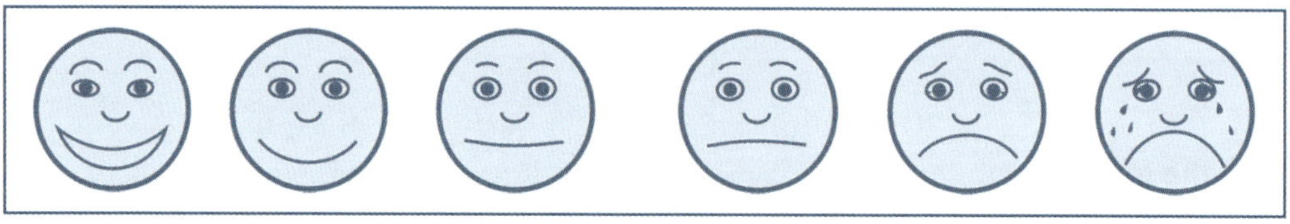

© C.K.

An older child can be trained to use the following scale from 0-10, where zero is no pain and ten is the worst pain he or she can imagine.

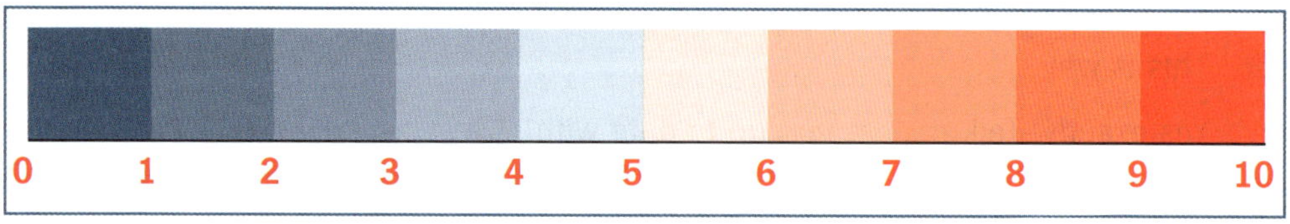

Imagine a dialogue between a nurse and a child. Ask him/her how much it hurts. Use the scale above.

GRAMMAR

Pronoms relatifs

• Emploi

Les pronoms relatifs permettent de relier deux propositions, évitant ainsi la répétition du nom qu'il représente : The patient who is in this room is very ill.

• Construction

Who (qui)	Pour un antécédent humain	The nurse who takes care of my father is very professional.
Where (où)	Pour un antécédent représentant un lieu	The hospital where I work is far.
Whose (dont)	Pour indiquer la possession (antécédent humain ou non humain)	Tomorrow we will operate on a boy whose forearm was badly burnt in a fire. That's the patient whose father works in paediatrics.
Which (ce qui/ce que)	Pour résumer la proposition précédente	I found him alone, which surprised me.
What (ce qui/ce que)	Pour introduire une proposition	He didn't know what he wanted.

Exercice 7

Réponse p. 152

Complétez les phrases suivantes avec *what* ou *which*.

1. He couldn't hear .... I was saying to him because he was deaf.
2. She doesn't take me seriously, ... irritates me.
3. Three nurses were absent, ... forced the ward sister to change the schedule.
4. She didn't know .... to think about his behaviour.
5. He drinks too much, ... is bad for his health.

Exercice 8

Réponse p. 152

Complétez les phrases suivantes en utilisant *which* ou *who*.

1. The medical dictionary .... is in our ward is very useful.
2. His father, ... is a well known surgeon, lives in the same city as us.
3. Cells, ... are the basic units of life, can be seen through a microscope.
4. You have worked in a hospital in Bordeaux and in Angoulême. .... one do you like best?
5. The specialist, ... treats me, is extremely competent.

Exercice 9

Réponse p. 153

Associez un élément de chaque colonne afin de composer des phrases cohérentes.

1. The two patients............ •	• .....A. whose anaesthetists were on strike, didn't perform the operation.
2. Those are the children..... •	• .....B. whose mothers were alcoholics.
3. The surgeon.................... •	• .....C. whose legs are broken, arrived yesterday.
4. He's the man.................. •	• .....D. whose daughter refused an abortion.

Exercice 10

Réponse p. 153

Complétez les phrases après avoir choisi la réponse correcte.

1. I know a child, ... mother took ecstasy during her pregnancy.
   whose; of whom; which
2. Hospital laboratories, ... goal is to identify the cause of infectious diseases, are more effective. *which; (ø); whose*
3. The E.N.T specialist .... I'm talking about, is my uncle. *of which; which; (ø)*
4. The people injured in the car accident, ... died yesterday, were my cousins.
   whose two; two of whom; two of which
5. The intern, ... wife is pregnant, is extremely competent.
   whose the; whose; of whom

Exercice 11

Réponse p. 153

Associez les éléments de chaque colonne afin de composer des phrases cohérentes.

1. A vaccine is a sterile medium.... •	• .... **A.** why he had an infection is obvious.
2. The reason............................ •	• .... **B.** when he met her.
3. The day.................................. •	• .... **C.** which contains a specific pathogen.
4. The nurses............................. •	• .... **D.** (that) the intern told us was true.
5. Everything.............................. •	• .... **E.** who(m) he works with are extremely competent.

Piste 50

Exercice 12

Réponse p. 153

Écoutez, puis répétez. Complétez la légende à l'aide des mots suivants :

- brain
- cerebellum
- spinal cord
- medulla

The brain

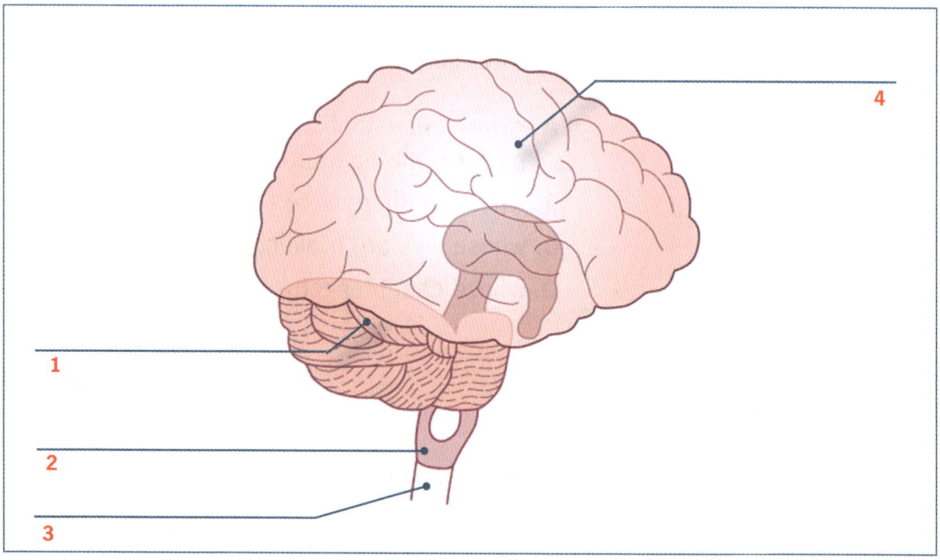

© A.C.R

https://www.lienmini.fr/angsoin19

Exercice 13 : Testez-vous !

Réponse p. 153

Traduisez en anglais.

1. S'il avait respecté le secret professionnel, elle n'aurait pas eu à faire face à ce conflit. ...
....
2. Vous n'auriez pas dû manger avant l'opération. ....
....
3. S'il n'avait pas été hospitalisé jeudi dernier, il aurait pu mourir. ....
....
4. Il aurait dû me le demander et je lui aurais donné ses antibiotiques. ....
....
5. Si vous aviez pris ces cachets, vous vous seriez senti beaucoup mieux. ....
....
6. Vous devez utiliser des gants jetables, ce qui réduit le risque d'infection. ....
....
7. Elle sait ce que tu devrais faire : vérifier sa tension toutes les trois heures. ....
....

Exercice 14 : Patient education

Réponse p. 153

Childhood asthma education

Cochez la (les) bonne(s) affirmation(s).

	True	False
1. Explain that asthma is not a long-term illness that is still there even when the child does not have any symptoms at the moment.		
2. Explain the causes of wheezing* and breathlessness*.		
3. Explain warning signs that mean the child needs to take medication, needs a doctor, or needs emergency care.		
4. Mention some common factors that can trigger* children's asthma (ex : colds, exercise, allergens, tobacco smoke.)		
5. Do not provide advice on triggers that can be avoided*.		

To help you

- **wheezing:** sifflement
- **breathlessness:** essoufflement
- **to trigger:** déclencher
- **to avoid:** éviter

https://www.lienmini.fr/angsoinq10a

Vocabulary quiz: Paediatric ward

Réponse p. 154

Complétez chaque définition avec le terme correct.

1. An .... is a piece of equipment which new babies are placed in when they are born too early.
a) bedroom **b)** ward **c)** incubator **d)** unit

2. I'll change her ...., it's all wet.
a) nappy **b)** dummy **c)** vaccination **d)** teddy bear

3. A .... helps your baby to rest easy and get to sleep in a timely manner.
a) furniture **b)** nappy **c)** ball **d)** comfort blanket

4. A .... is used to give milk to a baby.
a) spoon **b)** glass **c)** bottle **d)** plate

5. A rubber or plastic object for a baby to suck is called a ....
a) potty **b)** dummy **c)** sweet **d)** lolly

https://www.lienmini.fr/angsoinq10b

Vocabulary quiz: Pain in children & childhood diseases

Réponse p. 154

Complétez chaque définition avec le terme correct.

1. A face .... is used in order to assess* pain in children.
a) thermometer **b)** scale **c)** object **d)** thing

2. Children can communicate their .... by pointing to one of the faces.
a) joy **b)** emotion **c)** pain **d)** feeling

3. The disease that causes a slight fever and many spots on the skin is called ....
a) meningitis **b)** polio **c)** mumps **d)** chickenpox

4. The disease that causes painful swellings* in the neck is called ....
a) mumps **b)** ear infection **c)** measles **d)** rubella

5. He keeps on scratching his ear because of his ....
a) pain **b)** vaccination **c)** ear infection **d)** meningitis

To help you

- **to assess:** évaluer
- **swelling:** gonflement

Medical Vocabulary: unit 10

- **disease:** maladie
- **joint:** articulation
- **chickenpox:** varicelle
- **mumps:** oreillons
- **patient confidentiality:** secret professionnel
- **measles:** rougeole
- **nappy:** couche
- **spleen:** rate
- **brain:** cerveau

Let's discuss!

Professional skills and qualities

What are the professional skills and qualities needed to become a responsible nurse?

Corrigés

Exercice 1

1. If I knew her name I **would introduce** you.
2. If he had arrived earlier you **would have met** him.
3. He told her he would type this letter as soon as he **had** the information.
4. I **would operate** on you if it was possible.
5. If you had arrived on time I **could have done** it this morning.

Exercice 2

1. I would travel if I **had** enough time.
2. If I see Denis I **will give** him the medical report.
3. If I had known I **would have invited** them.
4. If he **had known** what was going to happen, he **would have done** something about it.
5. We **will stop** his treatment if he feels better.

Exercice 3

1. **Diseases**: breast
2. **Parts of the head**: hip
3. **Joints**: cheek
4. **Eye**: flu
5. **Bones**: cornea
6. **Organs**: toe

Exercice 4

1. diphtérie : diphtheria
2. rougeole : measles
3. rubéole : rubella/German measles
4. méningite : meningitis
5. varicelle : chickenpox
6. oreillons : mumps
7. otite : ear infection
8. poliomyélite : polio
9. coqueluche : whooping cough

Exercice 5

1. Incubator
2. Bottle
3. Nappy
4. Teddy bear
5. Dummy
6. Comfort blanket
7. Potty
8. Teat

Exercice 6

1. ... we have to keep your little baby in...
2. ... he keeps on scratching his left ear.
3. ... all his vaccinations?
4. ... is fond of his comfort-blanket.
5. What's his sleeping pattern like?
6. I'll change your nappy...

Exercice 7

1. He couldn't hear **what** I was saying to him because he was deaf.
2. She doesn't take me seriously, **which** irritates me.
3. Three nurses were absent, **which** forced the ward sister to change the schedule.
4. She didn't know **what** to think about his behaviour.
5. He drinks too much, **which** is bad for his health.

Exercice 8

1. The medical dictionary **which** is in our ward is very useful.
2. His father, **who** is a well known surgeon, lives in the same city as us.
3. Cells, **which** are the basic units of life, can be seen through a microscope.
4. You have worked in a hospital in Bordeaux and in Angoulême. **Which** one do you like best?

Corrigés

Exercice 9

1. The two patients............	.....**A.** whose anaesthetists were on strike, didn't perform the operation.
2. Those are the children.....	.....**B.** whose mothers were alcoholics.
3. The surgeon....................	.....**C.** whose legs are broken, arrived yesterday.
4. He's the man.....................	.....**D.** whose daughter refused an abortion.

Exercice 10

1. I know a child, **whose** mother took ecstasy during her pregnancy.
2. Hospital laboratories, **whose** goal is to identify the cause of infectious diseases, are more effective.
3. The E.N.T specialist **ø**. I'm talking about, is my uncle.
4. The people injured in the car accident, **two of whom** died yesterday, were my cousins.
5. The intern, **whose** wife is pregnant, is extremely competent.

Exercice 11

1. A vaccine is a sterile medium....	........**A.** why he had an infection is obvious.
2. The reason.............................	........**B.** when he met her.
3. The day.................................	........**C.** which contains a specific pathogen.
4. The nurses.............................	........**D.** (that) the intern told us was true.
5. Everything..............................	........**E.** who(m) he works with are extremely competent.

Exercice 12

1. Cerebellum **2.** Spinal cord **3.** Medulla **4.** Brain

Exercice 13 : Testez-vous !

1. If he had respected patient confidentiality, she wouldn't have to deal with this conflict.
2. You shouldn't have eaten before the operation.
3. If he hadn't been hospitalised last Thursday, he could have died.
4. He should have asked me and I would have given him his antibiotics.
5. If you had taken these pills/tablets you would have felt much better.
6. You have to use disposable gloves, which reduces the risk of infection.
7. She knows what you should do: check his blood pressure every three hours.

Exercice 14

1. False **2.** True **3.** True **4.** True **5.** False

Corrigés

Vocabulary quiz: Paediatric ward

1. incubator 2. nappy 3. comfort blanket 4. bottle 5. dummy

Vocabulary quiz: Pain in children & childhood diseases

1. scale 2. pain 3. chickenpox 4. mumps 5. ear infection

UNIT 11

UNIT 11

Carrying out a handover*

Toutes les pistes audio de l'unité à télécharger ici
https://www.lienmini.fr/angsoinu11

Piste 51

Dialogue between Mary and Pascale, Mr Brown and the nurse

Traduction p. 216

Listen to the dialogue. Pascale is handing over* to Mary. Mary's shift* is from 12:00 am to 8:00 pm.

Mary Have you had a busy morning?

Pascale Same as usual. I've talked about Mr Brown's discharge* with the surgeon. We'll discharge him next Friday. I didn't have time to talk to him about it. Can you speak to him?

Mary Certainly. I'll tell him to get in touch* with a District nurse. As you know, he has been on insulin since the beginning of his hospitalization. I'll pass on this information to his wife.

Pascale OK. Let me tell you about Mrs Favre in room 14, she doesn't feel as well today as yesterday. Her temperature seems higher. I've called Dr Lavau. He told me he would look in* at about 6:00.

Mary What about Mr Tournier?

Pascale Well, Dr Rainac thinks it's necessary to carry out* a certain number of tests. He suspects hepatitis B, but he wants to wait for the results of the tests to confirm his suspicions. Could you make sure that his lab reports are ready when he comes at 5:00?

Mary Sure.

In Mr Brown's room.

Nurse Good afternoon Mr Brown. So you're leaving next Friday?

Mr Brown Yes, I am. I wanted to apologize for my friend. He was rather rude the other day. He takes things too far!

Nurse Don't worry. Everything worked out* in the end.

Mr Brown Thank you very much for your help. I can't tell you how much I've appreciated your kindness during my stay. And thank you for speaking English to me. It was really reassuring.

Nurse Not at all. Have a good trip home! Bye!

To help you

- **to carry out a handover:** passer les transmissions
- **shift:** garde
- **discharge:** sortie
- **to get in touch:** prendre contact
- **to look in:** passer (voir quelqu'un brièvement)
- **to carry out:** effectuer (analyse/ recherche)
- **everything worked out:** tout s'est arrangé

Questions sur le dialogue

1. What does Mary have to pass on to Mrs Brown? ....

2. What does she need to prepare for Dr Rainac? ....

3. Why does Mr Brown apologize? ....

4. How do you think this handover went? ....

GRAMMAR

Discours direct/discours indirect

• Emploi

Quand on reproduit textuellement les propos d'une personne, il s'agit du discours direct. On le désigne généralement par des guillemets.

Lorsqu'on répète la phrase afin d'éviter une citation, il s'agit du discours indirect.

• Construction

Quand on met un propos au discours indirect, il faut vérifier que les temps des verbes reflètent le changement de contexte :

Discours direct	Discours indirect
Present	Preterit
"I am overweight."	She said she was overweight.
Futur	Conditional
"I will contact you as soon as possible."	He said he would contact me as soon as possible.
Preterit	Pluperfect
"He forgot to tell her."	She said he had forgotten to tell her.
Present perfect	Pluperfect
"I have never seen you before."	He said he had never seen me before.
Imperative	Infinitive
"Do your best to help him."	She told her to do her best to help him.

Exercice 1

Réponse p. 166

Transformez le discours direct en discours indirect.

1. "Did you take the prescription the intern gave you?", she asked him.
   She asked him if ....
2. The nurse: "How old are you?"
   The nurse asked me ....
3. "Don't panic" the doctor told him.
   The doctor told him ....
4. "You should exercise more" her nutritionist advised her.
   The nutritionist advised her ....
5. "I will telephone you when I receive the blood test", the doctor said.
   The doctor said ....
6. She asked him: "Have you ever visited our town?"
   She asked him if ....
7. The radiologist said: "I will contact you as soon as I've got your X-ray plates."
   The radiologist said ....

Exercice 2

Réponse p. 166

Transformez le discours indirect en discours direct.

1. He wondered if my father was on insulin.
   He asked me: " .... "
2. He asked me when she had her last dose.
   He asked me: " .... "
3. He asked me if she had any complications because of her diabetes.
   He asked me: " .... "
4. She asked us if Mary had had a heart attack before.
   She asked us: " .... "
5. She asked us if he had any other diseases.
   She asked us: " .... "
6. She asked me what my usual medication was.
   She asked us: " .... "

Travaillez à deux

A: You applied for a job as a nurse or auxiliary nurse for St Patrick's clinic a year ago.

This is what you were told about your job.

- pay rise after a year
- friendly environment
- prospects of training
- very close to a nursery school

After a year in the clinic you are really disappointed.

Everything you were told was wrong.

You want to speak to B, the senior registrar (chef de clinique).

A: start your complaints with:

You told me ....

You said that ....

B: answer A's complaints.

Piste 52

Exercice 3 : Disabilities

Réponse p. 166

Écoutez, puis répétez.

Complétez les phrases avec les mots suivants :

- bedridden
- blind
- deaf
- dumb[1]
- physically disabled

1. Helen can't speak, she is ....
2. Paul can't walk, he is ....
3. Joan can't hear, she is ....
4. Andrew can't see, he is ....
5. Walter can't get out of bed, he is ....

Piste 53

Exercice 4 : At the gynaecologist's

Traduction pp. 216-217
Réponse p. 166

Écoutez le dialogue et complétez la conversation entre le gynécologue et sa patiente. Utilisez les phrases suivantes :

- ... I had a miscarriage* three years ago.
- How many days does it last?
- ... did you begin to menstruate?
- Mostly the first day....

Doctor At what age **(1)** ....

Patient I was 15.

Doctor Tell me, when did you have your last period*?

Patient 14th August.

Doctor **(2)** ....

Patient Well, most of the time five or six days.

Doctor And do you have any pain with your periods?

Patient **(3)** .... but it's all right afterwards.

Doctor Do you have regular periods?

Patient Yes, I do usually.

Doctor How many times have you been pregnant*?

Patient Twice, but **(4)** ....

Doctor Did you have any trouble with your deliveries*?

Patient I had my son prematurely at seven months. And for my daughter, I had a Caesarean.

Doctor Thank you very much. Now, could you please lie down on the couch*.

To help you

- **miscarriage:** fausse couche
- **period(s):** règles
- **pregnant:** enceinte
- **delivery:** accouchement
- **couch:** table d'examen

Piste 54

Exercice 5 : Forms of contraception

Réponse p. 166

Écoutez.
Puis complétez le tableau suivant avec les équivalents anglais.

Spermicide	....
Stérilet (DIU)	....
Préservatif	....
Pilule	....
Abstinence périodique	....
Diaphragme	....

Travaillez à deux

Think of an event that happened yesterday in the hospital (the geriatric ward was on fire, for example).

A: You are one of the witnesses (a nurse, a doctor, a patient...).
Imagine the background to the story in detail.

B: As a journalist, you are going to interview **A** who witnessed the event.
You want to get information: *a)* about the past events. *b)* what is happening now. *c)* about the possible future events.

Exercice 6

Réponse p. 166

Écrivez la question qui permet d'obtenir l'information en bleu.

1. The HIV virus was discovered **in the mid 1980's**.
....
2. **Mrs Gate** had a smear test last week.
....
3. **A mother's risk of transmitting HIV to her child** can be reduced significantly.
....
4. The doctor will phone us **when he has received the results**.
....
5. He goes to the hospital **twice a month** to visit his father-in-law.
....

Exercice 7

Réponse p. 166

Complétez les phrases suivantes avec les prépositions *for, on, in* ou *from*.

1. How much money did you spend .... her education?
2. She was looking .... the bedpan.
3. The nurse is responsible .... her patients.
4. He is nice today. It depends .... his mood.
5. Could you fill .... these forms as soon as possible ? Thank you.
6. He is interested .... biology.
7. Your room is different .... mine. It's much bigger.
8. Thank you .... coming!
9. .... average, his results are not as good as we were expecting.
10. One .... five people is allergic to this antibiotic.

GRAMMAR

Comment traduire « faire faire »

L'expression « faire faire » peut s'exprimer de différentes manières.

Emploi	Construction	Exemple
Quand le verbe qui suit « faire » a un sens passif	Sujet + make + complément d'objet + infinitif sans "to"	He makes me laugh.
Quand le verbe qui suit « faire » a un sens actif	Sujet + have/get + complément d'objet + participe passé	He has/gets his car repaired once a year.

Exercice 8

Réponse p. 167

Complétez les phrases avec *make, made* ou *have, had*.

1. The dermatologist told her to .... her wart removed.
2. He hopes this pill won't .... him too sleepy.
3. Last Wednesday, the doctor .... me wait for an hour. I was furious!
4. The nurse .... him take his medicine even though he didn't want to.
5. You........................ me laugh!
6. I .... my hair cut a month ago.
7. Yesterday, the low temperature .... all the patients shiver.

Exercice 9

Réponse p. 167

« Faire » peut se traduire autrement que par *make* ou *have*. Traduisez les expressions ci-dessous, puis employez-les dans des phrases.

1. Faire venir le médecin : ....

   ....
2. Faire visiter quelque chose à quelqu'un : ....

   ....
3. Faire entrer quelqu'un : ....

   ....
4. Faire remarquer quelque chose : ....

   ....

Piste 55 Exercice 10

Réponse p. 167

Écoutez, puis répétez. Complétez la légende à l'aide des mots suivants :

- ovary
- uterine tube
- vagina
- womb/uterus
- cervix uteri

Female reproductive system

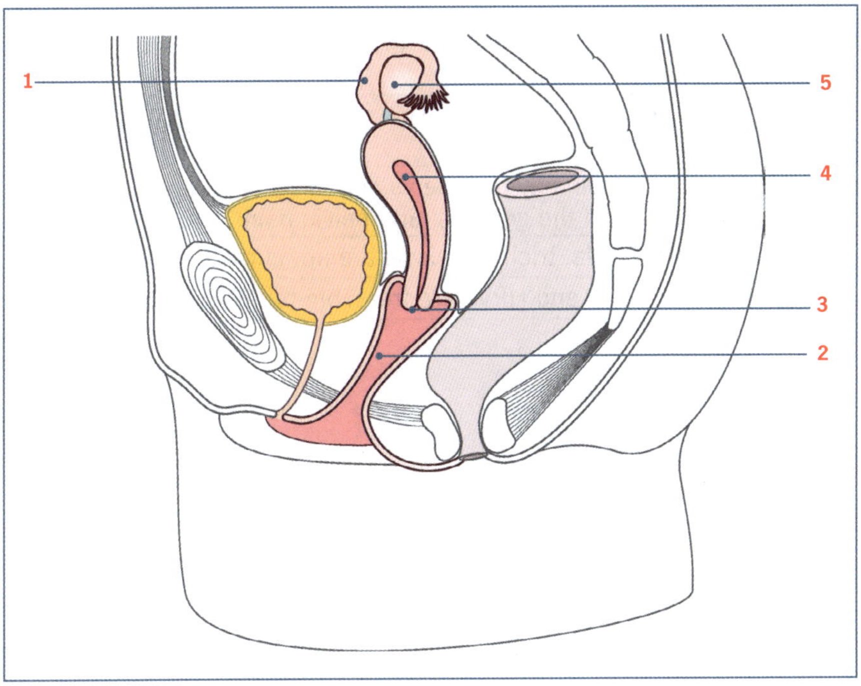

© S.M.

https://www.lienmini.fr/angsoin20

Exercice 11 : Testez-vous !

Réponse p. 167

Traduisez en anglais.

1. Il lui a demandé à quelle heure elle avait passé les transmissions à l'obstétricien. ....
2. Je vous recommande de ne pas le contacter avant d'avoir ses clichés-radio. ....
3. Elle nous a dit qu'il était alité depuis plus d'une semaine. ....
4. Il s'intéresse beaucoup à la bactériologie et il est responsable de ce laboratoire depuis mars. ....
5. Le gynécologue lui a dit de se faire enlever l'ovaire gauche. ....
6. Elle est enceinte de sept mois. J'ai bien peur qu'elle accouche d'un prématuré. ....
7. Elle avait tellement mal à la gorge qu'elle a fait venir le médecin. ....

Exercice 12 : Patient information

Réponse p. 167

Sexually transmitted infections (STI) or Sexually transmitted diseases (STD)

Cochez la (les) bonne(s) affirmation(s).

	True	False
1. STI or STD are infections that are commonly spread by sex, especially vaginal intercourse, anal sex or oral sex.		
2. Most STIs initially do not cause symptoms. This results in a greater risk of passing the disease on to others.		
3. Symptoms and signs of disease may include vaginal discharge, penile discharge, ulcers on or around the genitals, and pelvic pain.		
4. Syphilis, gonorrhea*, chlamydia, trichomoniasis are not curable.		
5. Herpes, hepatitis B, HIV/AIDS, and HPV* are treatable but not curable.		

To help you

- **gonorrhea:** blennorragie
- **HPV:** human papillomavirus

https://www.lienmini.fr/angsoinq11

Verbs quiz: Carrying out a handover

Réponse p. 167

Complétez chaque affirmation avec le verbe correct.

1. After his discharge he will have to .... with a district nurse.
a) speak **b)** phone **c)** get in touch **d)** call

2. We suspect hepatitis B, so it is necessary to .... a certain number of tests.
a) go on **b)** carry out **c)** make **d)** start

3. After his shift from 6:00 am to 1:00 pm he has to .... to Carol.
a) hand on **b)** hand out **c)** hand over **d)** hand in

4. She'll .... this information to the patient as soon as possible.
a) pass on **b)** do **c)** take **d)** pass in

5. They didn't have the time to .... the patient about her discharge*.
a) go **b)** talk to **c)** deal **d)** work

https://www.lienmini.fr/angsoinq11b

Vocabulary quiz: Forms of contraception

Réponse p. 167

Complétez chaque définition avec le terme correct.

1. Another word for Intra uterine Device (IUD) is ....

a) pill **b)** diaphragm **c)** coil **d)** condom

2. The substance that kills sperm, used during sex to prevent the woman form becoming pregnant is called ....

a) condom **b)** implant **c)** pill **d)** spermicide

3. People sometimes call it « .... ». But you don't have to wait until the morning after sex to take it. In fact, it is more effective the sooner you take.

a) IUD **b)** pill **c)** coil **d)** morning-after pill

4. The contraceptive.. releases* the hormone progestogen into your bloodstream to prevent pregnancy and lasts for 3 years.

a) cervix **b)** condom
c) implant **d)** periodic abstinence

5. A .... is the form of birth control that is a shallow cup shaped* like a little saucer* made of soft silicone.

a) diaphragm **b)** womb
c) IUD **d)** spermicide

To help you

- **discharge:** sortie
- **to release:** libérer
- **shallow:** peu profonde
- **shaped like:** qui a la forme de
- **saucer:** coupelle

Medical Vocabulary: unit 11

- **to carry out a handover:** passer les transmissions
- **X-ray plate:** cliché radiologique
- **bedridden:** alité
- **disability:** infirmité
- **miscarriage:** fausse couche
- **coil/IUD (intra-uterine device):** stérilet
- **shift:** garde
- **smear test:** frottis
- **pregnant:** enceinte
- **cervix:** col de l'utérus
- **womb:** utérus

Let's discuss!

Contraception

There are roughly 200.000 abortions a year in France. Many of these abortions are carried out because women have forgotten take the pill.

Why are abortions carried out so frequently, when there are many forms of contraception?

What should the role of the school nurse be regarding information and education about contraception?

Corrigés

Exercice 1

1. She asked him if **he had taken the prescription the intern had given him**.
2. The nurse asked me **how old I was**.
3. The doctor told him **not to panic**.
4. The nutritionist advised her **to exercise more**.
5. The doctor said **he would telephone me when he received the blood test**.
6. She asked him if **he had ever visited their town**.
7. The radiologist said **he would contact me as soon as he got my X-ray plates**.

Exercice 2

1. Is your father on insulin?
2. When did she have her last dose?
3. Has she got any complications because of her diabetes?
4. Has she had a heart attack before?
5. Has he got any other diseases?
6. What is your usual medication?

Exercice 3

1. dumb
2. physically disabled
3. deaf
4. blind
5. bedridden.

Exercice 4

1. ... did you begin to menstruate?
2. How many days does it last?
3. Mostly the first day...
4. ... I had a miscarriage three years ago.

Exercice 5

Spermicide	**Spermicide**
Stérilet (DIU)	**Coil / Intra Uterine Device (IUD)**
Préservatif	**Condom**
Pilule	**Pill**
Abstinence périodique	**Periodic abstinence** **Rhythm method**
Diaphragme	**Diaphragm**

Exercice 6

1. When was the HIV virus discovered?
2. Who had a smear test last week?
3. Which risks can be reduced significantly?
4. When will he/the doctor phone us?
5. How often does he go to the hospital?

Exercice 7

1. How much money did you spend **on** her education?
2. She was looking **for** the bedpan.
3. The nurse is responsible **for** her patients.
4. He is nice today. It depends **on** his mood.
5. Could you fill **in** these forms as soon as possible ? Thank you.
6. He is interested **in** biology.
7. Your room is different **from** mine. It's much bigger.
8. Thank you **for** coming!
9. **On** average, his results are not as good as we were expecting.
10. One **in** five people is allergic to this antibiotic.

Corrigés

Exercice 8

1. The dermatologist told her to **have** her wart removed.
2. He hopes this pill won't **make** him too sleepy.
3. Last Wednesday, the doctor **made** me wait for an hour. I was furious!
4. The nurse **made** him take his medicine even though he didn't want to.
5. You **make** me laugh!
6. I **had** my hair cut a month ago.
7. Yesterday, the low temperature **made** all the patients shiver.

Exercice 9

1. to call/to send for the doctor
2. to show somebody around
3. to show somebody in
4. to point out/to remark/to notice something

Exercice 10

1. uterine tube
2. vagina
3. cervix uteri
4. womb/uterus
5. ovary

Exercice 11 : Testez-vous !

1. He asked her what time she had passed on the reports to the obstetrician.
2. I recommend that you do not contact him before getting his X-ray plates.
3. She told us he had been bedridden for more than a week.
4. He is really interested in bacteriology and he has been in charge of this lab since March.
5. The gynaecologist (Brit)/gynecologist (US) told her to have her left ovary removed.
6. She is seven months pregnant. I'm afraid she'll give birth prematurely.
7. She had such a sore throat (that) she called/sent for the doctor.

Exercice 12

1. True
2. True
3. True
4. False
5. True

Verbs quiz: Carrying out a handover

1. get in touch
2. carry out
3. hand over
4. pass on
5. talk to

Vocabulary quiz: Forms of contraception

1. coil
2. spermicide
3. morning-after pill
4. implant
5. diaphragm

UNIT 12

UNIT 12 Visiting a diabetic patient at home

Toutes les pistes audio de l'unité à télécharger ici
https://www.lienmini.fr/angsoinu12

Piste 56 Dialogue between Mr Brown and the nurse

Traduction p. 217

Listen to the dialogue. Mr Brown is now at home. His District nurse* is talking to him.

Nurse Good morning Mr Brown. I'm glad to see you back home. I was told you had some complications when you were in hospital.

Mr Brown Yes I did, indeed. I had a difficult time, actually. I had a pulmonary embolism.

Nurse How do you feel now?

Mr Brown Well, of course, I feel much better. You know, I gave up smoking and I firmly intend to* keep to my diet. By the way, I need some advice about it, I am not quite clear* about what I should do.

Nurse No problem. Anyway, we have plenty of time. Let me just read your prescription* again. OK, so I have to change your dressing everyday and take a blood sample every evening.

Mr Brown And what about my diabetes?

Nurse I'll show you how to check your blood sugar level* and how to take your insulin. For the first few days, we'll do it together, then, you'll be able to do it by yourself*.

Mr Brown I was told it was very difficult to do it by yourself.

Nurse No, don't worry. The new techniques are easier today. What is difficult is to adapt the insulin doses to your blood sugar level. But you know, you'll manage the situation very well*.

Mr Brown OK. What time will you come for my injection tomorrow?

Nurse I'd say around 7:30 am. I'll do your dressing as well. I'm sure you'll soon be better. See you tomorrow.

Mr Brown Bye bye, see you tomorrow.

To help you

- **district/visiting/home nurse:** infirmière à domicile/libérale
- **I firmly intend to:** j'ai fermement l'intention
- **I am not quite clear:** je n'ai pas très bien saisi
- **prescription:** ordonnance
- **blood sugar level:** glycémie
- **by yourself:** tout seul
- **you'll manage the situation very well:** vous vous en sortirez très bien

Questions sur le dialogue

1. How does the district nurse know about Mr Brown's complications? ....
2. What does Mr Brown intend to do? ....
3. What does the nurse have to do everyday? ....
4. How do you think this visit went? ....

GRAMMAR

Le passif

• Emploi

La forme passive est employée :

– pour traduire un passif français :

. He will be anaesthetized.

. The operation is being carried out by Dr Barber: L'opération est faite par le docteur Barber.

– pour traduire « on » :

. I was told: On m'a dit.

. English is spoken here: On parle anglais ici.

– quand un verbe a deux compléments : He was sent several emails: On lui a envoyé plusieurs e-mails.

• Construction

Le passif est formé de : to be (conjugué) + participe passé.

Temps	Exemple
Présent simple	X-rays are taken everyday.
Présent continu	X-rays are being taken now.
Futur	X-rays will be taken tomorrow.
Conditionnel	X-rays would be taken if we could.
Prétérit	X-rays were taken yesterday.
Plus-perfect	X-rays had been taken the day before.

Exercice 1

Réponse p. 182

Mettez les phrases suivantes au passif.

1. They detected many polyps.
Many polyps ....
2. Fleming discovered penicillin in the early 20th century.
Penicillin ....
3. He discovered the AIDS virus in 1984.
The AIDS virus ....
4. The Red Cross will help the starving population.
The starving population ....
5. Florey tested penicillin on a patient in the early 1940s.
Penicillin ....

Exercice 2

Réponse p. 182

Faites cinq phrases en utilisant un élément dans chaque colonne.

This test	will be provided	on our ward.
You	is said	four pills a day.
I	told me	to use your computer.
She	was given	to be a good GP.
They	is performed	with the food they need.

1. ....
2. ....
3. ....
4. ....
5. ....

Piste 57

Exercice 3

Réponse p. 182

Écoutez, puis répétez.

À chaque mot sa définition.

• hip • knee • wrist • ankle • neck • toe

1. The joint connecting the foot with the leg: ....
2. The upper part of the thighbone on each side of the body: ....
3. The joint between the thigh and the lower leg: ....
4. The part of the body that connects the head with the shoulders: ....
5. One of five terminal members of the foot: ....
6. The joint connecting the hand with the forearm: ....

Piste 58

Exercice 4

Réponse p. 182

Écoutez les phrases, puis complétez-les.

1. She thought that she was .... about her diet. In a way, she was: ...., lots of fish, plenty of fruit and vegetables. The only problem is ....
2. She .... other risk factors: tobacco, high salt and a ....
3. Her GP recommended her to .... for high blood pressure at least once a year.
4. .... is essential to avoid the risk of major cardiovascular damage, stroke and ....

Travaillez à deux

People say that we will soon be able to consult the doctor from home, for instance via the Internet.

What do you think about this idea?

In your opinion, what are the advantages and disadvantages? Discuss.

Piste 59

Exercice 5 : At the dermatologist's

Traduction p. 218

Réponse p. 182

Écoutez le dialogue et complétez la conversation entre le dermatologue et le patient. Utilisez les phrases suivantes :

- Is it itching*?
- … this rash*…
- … rather than itches.
- It may take several weeks.
- … when the shingles* is localized in this area.
- … it must be what we call shingles.

Patient I've got **(1)** .... on my back and it's all red.

Doctor Since when?

Patient It started three days ago.

Doctor **(2)** ....

Patient Yes, it is but I'd say it burns **(3)** ....

....

Doctor Have you ever had this type of rash* before?

Patient No, this is the first time.

Doctor Let's have a look. Oh, I see, **(4)** ....

....

Patient Is it serious?

Doctor Well, no. Not so much when **(5)** ....
But it's difficult to cure it. **(6)** ....
You'll have to be patient.

Patient I see. All right... My wife will come and see you tomorrow: her eczema is back again.

To help you

- **Is it itching?:** avez-vous des démangeaisons ?/est-ce que ça vous gratte ?
- **rash:** rougeur/éruption
- **shingles:** zona

Piste 60

Exercice 6

Réponse p. 182

Écoutez et complétez la légende à l'aide des mots suivants :

- prostate
- urinary bladder
- testicle
- penis
- urethra
- scrotum

Male reproductive system

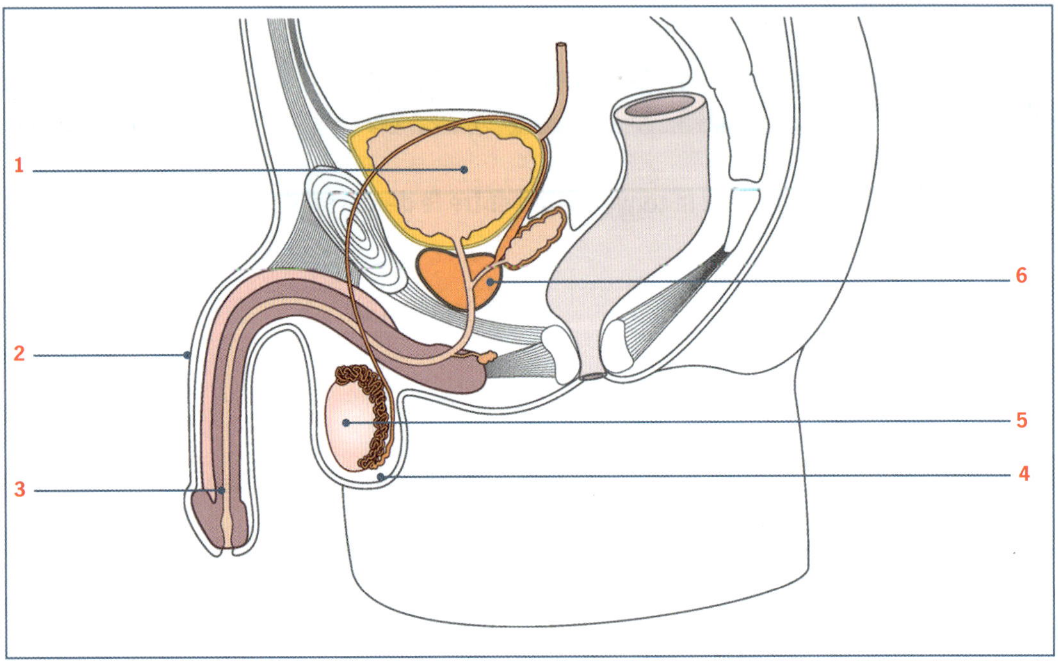

© S.M.

https://www.lienmini.fr/angsoin21

Piste 61

Exercice 7 : Decontamination

Réponse p. 182

Écoutez les consignes, puis réécrivez-les dans le bon ordre.

1. Brush the instruments and rinse them.
2. Put the disinfectant solution into the water.
3. Dip the instruments into the germicidal solution. Wait for 10 minutes.
4. Wipe them with a clean towel and proceed to sterilization.

1. ....
2. ....
3. ....
4. ....

Piste 62 — Travaillez à deux : Disinfection and sterilization

To prevent the transmission of microbial diseases, medical instruments and equipment used for care must be disinfected and sterilized.

In your opinion, what are the advantages and disadvantages of these means of disinfection and sterilization?

1. Dry heat sterilization.
2. Micro-wave sterilization.
3. Ethylene oxide sterilization.
4. Autoclaving sterilization.
5. Ultraviolet ray sterilization.

Exercice 8 : Révision générale

Réponse p. 182

Dans chaque phrase, conjuguez le verbe selon le temps approprié au contexte.

1. I .... (*to be*) very happy when the operation is finished.
2. "– What .... you (*to do*) last night?" – "I .... (*to stay*) at home because I have an exam today."
3. We .... (*to call*) his family yesterday.
4. The teacher told us .... (*to come*) early.
5. When the children .... (*to eat*) their lunch, their parents left the day-nursery.
6. If I had known, I .... (*to spend*) more time with my patients.
7. I .... (*to watch*) TV when the nurse came into my room to give me my medication.
8. Today I never .... (*to think*) about my illness.
9. I .... (*to enjoy*) my holidays if I had not been allergic to this antibiotic.
10. When I have enough time, I .... (*to write*) my journal abstract; in two days or so.
11. Our GP .... (*to go*) to England every year.
12. Have you ever .... (*to see*) a scar like that?
13. The surgeon .... (*to operate*) now.
14. Last year, I .... (*to decide*) to become a nurse because it is a rewarding profession.

Exercice 9 : Testez-vous !

Réponse p. 183

Traduisez en anglais.

1. On m'a dit que ce virus serait isolé très bientôt. ....

2. On lui a envoyé toutes ses analyses sanguines, mais il ne les a pas encore reçues. ....

3. Tu n'es pas obligé d'essuyer les instruments maintenant, il nous reste un peu de temps. ....

4. Elle avait une plaque rouge sur le bras gauche depuis plusieurs jours. ....

5. L'infirmière libérale lui a dit : « N'hésitez pas à m'appeler si vous avez un problème. » ....

6. Il aurait pu stériliser quelques instruments avant de partir. ....

7. Le jour où il l'a rencontrée, elle lui a expliqué la raison pour laquelle elle avait eu une infection. ....

Exercice 10 : Patient education

Réponse p. 183

How to change a dressing

Cochez la (les) bonne(s) affirmation(s).

	True	False
1. You should have a clean work surface on which to place all equipment you will need. You may use a clean towel to cover your work surface.		
2. Never wash your hands with soap and water before touching the dressing.		
3. After removing the dressing, wrap* it in a plastic bag or paper towel before throwing it into the trash can*.		
4. Wash your hands with soap and water again after removing the old dressing. This prevents any germs on the old dressing from getting onto the clean dressing.		
5. Do not apply the clean dressing as directed* by your doctor or nurse.		

To help you

- **to wrap:** envelopper
- **trash can:** poubelle
- **to direct:** indiquer

Exercice 11 : Patient education in diabetes

Réponse p. 183

Associez la question à sa réponse.

1. What is diabetes exactly? •
2. What is insulin? •
3. What happens if it is not treated? •
4. What is Type 1 diabetes? •
5. What is Type 2 diabetes? •

- • A. A hormone produced in the pancreas, which regulates the amount of glucose in the blood.
- • B. High blood glucose can cause long-term complications.
- • C. It is a metabolic disease. The body is enable to produce any or enough insulin and that causes elevated levels of glucose in the blood.
- • D. The body becomes resistant to the effects of insulin and the pancreas may retain some ability to produce insulin.
- • E. Insulin production by the beta cells of the pancreas is impaired.

To help you

- **impaired:** affaibli, détérioré, diminué

Exercice 12 : Common symptoms of diabetes

Réponse p. 183

Écrivez les questions qui correspondent aux réponses du tableau ci-dessous.

1. What are the common symptoms of diabetes?
2. What are the signs of low blood sugar (hypoglycemia)?
3. What are the signs of high blood sugar (hyperglycemia)?

....	....	....
• Increased thirst • Headaches • Trouble concentrating • Blurred vision* • Frequent urination • Weight loss • Blood sugar more than 180 mg/dL • Risk of coma	• Sweating* (almost always present) • Nervousness • Shakiness* • Weakness* • Extreme hunger • Slight nausea • Dizziness* • Headache • Blurred vision • A fast heartbeat • Feeling anxious • Risk of coma	• Hunger • Urinating more often • Increased thirst • Dry mouth • Itching* • Blurred vision • Fatigue

To help you

- **blurred vision:** vision trouble
- **sweating:** sudation, transpiration
- **shakiness:** manque de stabilité
- **weakness:** (sensation de) fatigue
- **dizziness:** vertiges
- **itching:** démangeaison

Exercice 13 : Parts of an insulin pen

Réponse p. 183

Complétez la légende avec les mots suivants :

- dosage indicator
- insulin reservoir
- dose window
- pen cap
- dosage selector
- injection button

1. ....
2. ....
3. ....
4. ....
5. ....
6. ....

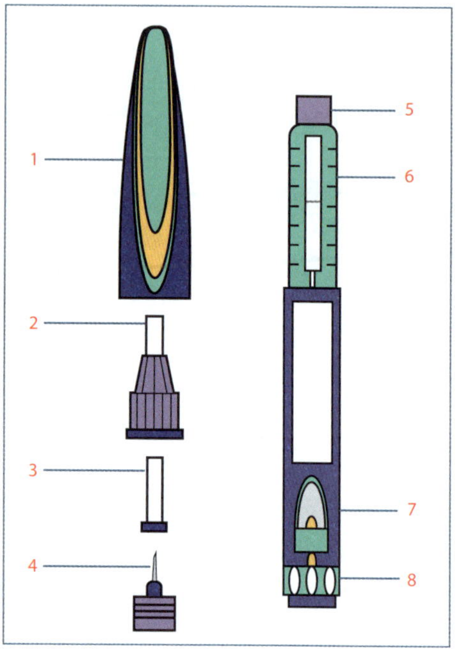

Puis, écrivez l'équivalent en anglais :

7. capuchon de stylo : ....
8. cartouche : ....
9. sélecteur de dose : ....
10. bouton poussoir : ....
11. fenêtre d'indication de la dose : ....
12. indicateur : ....

https://www.lienmini.fr/angsoin22

Exercice 14 : How to use an insulin pen

Réponse p. 184

Classez dans le bon ordre les indications du mode d'emploi du stylo à insuline en les numérotant de 1 à 11 au fil des trois grandes étapes d'utilisation A, B et C.

A.

.... Check the drug label to be sure it is what your doctor prescribed. Remove pen cap.
.... Roll the pen between your hands. You must also turn the pen up and down ten times.
.... Wash your hands.
.... Wipe* the tip* of the pen where the needle will attach with an alcohol swab.

B.

.... Decide where on your body you will give the shot. (The shot should be given in a different place each time. It depends on the type of insulin.)
.... Holding* the pen with the needle pointing upwards, press the button until* at least* a drop of insulin appears.
.... Insert the needle at a 90 degree angle.
.... Dial* the number of units you need to take.

C.

.... If you bleed* when the needle comes out, press gently with an alcohol swab on the skin immediately.

.... While keeping needle under skin, press the button all the way returning to zero, and keep pressing for six to ten seconds.

.... Carefully replace outer needle cap over.

To help you

- **to wipe:** essuyer
- **holding:** en tenant
- **until:** jusqu'à ce que
- **at least:** au moins
- **to bleed:** saigner
- **to dial:** sélectionner/composer
- **tip:** bout

Exercice 15 : Advantages of an insulin pen

Réponse p. 184

Cochez la (les) bonne(s) affirmation(s).

	True	False
1. Easy to use and carry		
2. No need to draw the insulin dose from a vial*/bottle		
3. Cannot contain different kinds of insulin together in a prescribed dose		
4. Doses can be easily dialed*		
5. To some people it may be less scary* than a syringe		
6. Can be used for most insulin types		

To help you

- **vial:** ampoule
- **scary:** effrayant
- **to dial:** (ici) faire

Exercice 16 : How a blood glucose meter work

Réponse p. 184

Écrivez la question au-dessus de la réponse qui lui correspond.

1. How does a blood glucose meter work?
2. How do I keep track*?
3. Why should I check?
4. When should I check?
5. Can exercise make my blood sugar levels* fluctuate?
6. How should I use a blood sugar meter?

A. It is a computerised device* that measures the amount of glucose from a sample of your blood and displays* it on a screen*.

B. You have to prick the side of your fingertip* with a small needle (lancet) to collect a drop of blood. Then, place the drop of blood on a special test strip inserted into your meter. Within one second the meter shows the results of your test.

C. Checking your blood sugar levels has many benefits. For example, if you test your blood sugar levels before and after meals this helps you see how eating certain foods affect those levels. So, you can adjust you food choices.

D. Yes, so test them regularly when you're active.

E. In general, most people with diabetes test their blood sugar levels before meals.

F. You have to write down the results in a log book*. This makes it easier for you and the nurse or the doctor to see the trends* in your blood sugar levels.

To help you

- **tract:** trace
- **level:** niveau/taux
- **device:** appareil
- **to display:** afficher
- **screen:** écran
- **fingertip:** bout du doigt
- **log book:** carnet
- **trend:** évolution/tendance

https://www.lienmini.fr/angsoinq12a

Vocabulary quiz: Medical equipment

Réponse p. 184

Complétez chaque définition avec le terme correct.

1. An .... is used to inject insulin for the treatment of diabetes.
a) pill box **b)** needle **c)** insulin pen **d)** dosage selector

2. A diabetic patient should write down his blood sugar level in a ....
a) log book **b)** exercice book **c)** screen **d)** device

3. A .... is a small, portable machine that is used to measure how much glucose is in the blood.
a) insulin pen **b)** tube **c)** needle **d)** blood glucose meter

4. A small container that pills are carried in is called .... or pillbox.
a) reservoir **b)** pill organiser **c)** dosage indicator **d)** dose window

5. A .... destroys microorganisms usually by bringing to a high temperature with steam, dry heat, or boiling liquid.
a) incubator **b)** splint **c)** sterilizer **d)** probe

https://www.lienmini.fr/angsoinq12b

Vocabulary quiz: Common symptoms of diabetes

Réponse p. 184

Complétez chaque définition avec le terme correct.

1. The primary symptom of .... is excessive amounts glucose in the urine.
a) hypoglycemia **b)** hyperglycemia **c)** rash **d)** infection

2. Other symptoms and signs of high blood sugar levels in the blood are .... , increased thirst and headaches.
a) stiffness **b)** hot flash **c)** insomnia **d)** blurred vision

3. The other common symptoms of diabetes is hunger, urinating more and ....
a) loss of libido **b)** increased thirst **c)** vaginal dryness **d)** night sweats

4. .... is a sensation of spinning around* and losing your balance*.
a) headache **b)** fatigue **c)** dizziness **d)** anxiety

5. .... is the uncomfortable feeling on your skin that makes you want to scratch*.
a) urinating **b)** itching **c)** crying **d)** shaking

To help you

- **to spin around:** tournoyer
- **balance:** équilibre
- **scratch :** se gratter

Medical Vocabulary: unit 12

- **AIDS:** SIDA
- **blood sugar level:** glycémie
- **waiting-room:** salle d'attente
- **home medical care:** soins à domicile
- **prescription:** ordonnance
- **to itch:** avoir des démangeaisons
- **toe:** orteil
- **thighbone:** fémur
- **blood test:** analyse sanguine

Let's discuss!

Home medical care

For some years, home medical care has become a priority for healthcare authorities.

What are the advantages and disadvantages of home care?

Corrigés

Exercice 1

1. Many polyps were detected.
2. Penicillin was discovered in the early 20th century by Fleming.
3. The AIDS virus was discovered in 1984.
4. The starving population will be helped by the Red Cross.
5. Penicillin was tested on a patient in the early 1940s by Florey.

Exercice 2

1. This test is performed on our ward.
2. You told me to use your computer.
3. I/She was given four pills a day.
4. She is said to be a good GP.
5. They/You will be provided with the food they need.

Exercice 3

1. ankle
2. hip
3. knee
4. neck
5. toe
6. wrist

Exercice 4

1. She thought that she was **careful** about her diet. In a way, she was: **low-fat**, lots of fish, plenty of fruit and vegetables. The only problem is **that she ate too much**.
2. She **combined** other risk factors: tobacco, high salt, a **sedentary life-style**.
3. Her GP recommended her to **be screened** for high blood pressure at least once a year.
4. **Early diagnosis** is essential to avoid the risk of major cardiovascular damage, stroke and **renal disorders**.

Exercice 5

1. ... this rash...
2. Is it itching?
3. ... rather than itches.
4. ... It must be what we call shingles.
5. ... the shingles is localised in this area.
6. It may take several weeks

Exercice 6

1. urinary bladder
2. penis
3. urethra
4. scrotum
5. testicle
6. prostate

Exercice 7

1. Put the disinfectant solution into the water.
2. Dip the instruments into the germicidal solution. Wait for 10 minutes.
3. Brush the instruments and rinse them.
4. Wipe them with a clean towel and proceed to sterilization.

Exercice 8 : Révision générale

1. I **will be** very happy when the operation is finished.
2. "– What **did** you **do** last night?" – "I **stayed** at home because I have an exam today."
3. We **called** his family yesterday.
4. The teacher told us **to come** early.
5. When the children **had eaten** their lunch, their parents left the day-nursery.
6. If I had known, I **would have spent** more time with my patients.
7. I **was watching** TV when the nurse came into my room to give me my medication.
8. Today I never **think** about my illness.
9. I **would have enjoyed** my holidays if I had not been allergic to this antibiotic.
10. When I have enough time, I **will write** my journal abstract; in two days or so.
11. Our GP **goes** to England every year.
12. Have you ever **seen** a scar like that?
13. The surgeon **is operating** now.
14. Last year, I **decided** to become a nurse because it is a rewarding profession.

Corrigés

Exercice 9 : Testez-vous !

1. I was told this virus would be isolated very soon.
2. He was sent all his blood tests, but he hasn't received them yet.
3. You needn't/don't have to wipe these instruments now, we have a little time left.
4. She had had a red rash on her left arm for several days.
5. The home/visiting/district nurse told him: "Don't hesitate to call me if you have a problem."
6. He could have sterilized a few instruments before leaving.
7. The day (when) he met her, she told him the reason why she had had an infection.

Exercice 10

1. True
2. False
3. True
4. True
5. False

Exercice 11

1. C
2. A
3. B
4. E
5. D

Exercice 12

What are the symptoms of high blood sugar (hyperglycemia)?	What are the symptoms of low blood sugar (hypoglycemia)?	What are the other common symptoms of diabetes?
• Increased thirst • Headaches • Trouble concentrating • Blurred vision* • Frequent urination • Weight loss • Blood sugar more than 180 mg/dL • Risk of coma	• Sweating* (almost always present) • Nervousness • Shakiness* • Weakness* • Extreme hunger • Slight nausea • Dizziness* • Headache • Blurred vision • A fast heartbeat • Feeling anxious • Risk of coma	• Hunger • Urinating more often • Increased thirst • Dry mouth • Itching* • Blurred vision • Fatigue

Exercice 13

1. pen cap
2. insulin reservoir
3. dose window
4. dosage indicator
5. injection button
6. dosage selector
7. capuchon du stylo : pen cap
8. cartouche : insulin reservoir
9. sélecteur de dose : dosage selector
10. bouton poussoir : injection button
11. fenêtre d'indication de dose : dose window
12. indicateur : dosage indicator

Corrigés

Exercice 14

A.

1. Wash your hands.
2. Check the drug label to be sure it is what your doctor prescribed. Remove pen cap.
3. Roll the pen between your hands. You must also turn the pen up and down ten times.
4. Wipe the tip of the pen where the needle will attach with an alcohol swab.

B.

5. Holding the pen with the needle pointing upwards, press the button until at least a drop of insulin appears.
6. Dial the number of units you need to take.
7. Decide where on your body you will give the shot. (The shot should be given in a different place each time. It depends on the type of insulin)
8. Insert the needle at a 90 degree angle.

C.

9. While keeping needle under skin, press the button all the way returning to zero, and keep pressing for six to ten seconds.
10. If you bleed when the needle comes out, press gently with an alcohol swab on the skin immediately.
11. Carefully replace outer needle cap over.

Exercice 15

1. True
2. True
3. False
4. True
5. True
6. True

Exercice 16

1. Réponse A
2. Réponse F
3. Réponse C
4. Réponse E
5. Réponse D
6. Réponse B

Vocabulary quiz: Medical equipment

1. insulin pen
2. log book
3. blood glucose meter
4. pill organiser
5. sterilizer

Vocabulary quiz: Common symptoms of diabetes

1. hyperglycemia
2. blurred vision
3. increased thirst
4. dizziness
5. itching

UNIT 13

UNIT 13 Palliative care

Dialogue between Mrs Wilson and the nurse

Traduction p. 218

A nurse is answering Mrs Wilson's questions about her mother's admission in palliative care.

Mrs Wilson Does palliative care mean that my mother is going to die?

Nurse Not necessarily. It's true that palliative care serves* many people with life-threatening* or terminal illnesses. But, you know, some patients are cured and no longer need palliative care.

Mrs Wilson Could you tell me what palliative care is exactly?

Nurse It is specialised medical care for patients living with a serious illness, like your mother. This type of care is focused on giving relief* from the symptoms and stress of the illness. The care team is here to improve your mother's quality of life and yours as well.

Mrs Wilson How long can my mother live with palliative care?

Nurse Usually less than six months. But your mother, even with a life expectancy* of a few years, can still choose a comfort-focused approach. She will get advice on pain and symptom control through consultation services.

Mrs Wilson How do you know when someone is ready for palliative care?

Nurse A decision to begin palliative care includes* many factors. Ideally the decision includes a discussion with the health care team. Some questions can help us determine when palliative care becomes necessary.

Mrs Wilson What are these questions about?

Nurse For example, what options are available for treatment? What does the person living with the illness want? What is the nature and the course of the illness?

Mrs Wilson Thank you very much for your answers.

Nurse Not at all.

To help you

- **to serve:** être au service de
- **life-threatening:** extrêmement grave
- **relief:** soulagement
- **life expectancy:** espérance de vie
- **to include:** comprendre, inclure, englober

Questions sur le dialogue

1. What is a palliative care? ....

....

....

2. How long can a patient live in palliative care? ....

....

....

3. What questions can help the medical and nursing staff determine when palliative care becomes necessary? ....

....

....

GRAMMAR

Mots de liaison

Deux phrases ou deux propositions peuvent être reliées par des mots de liaison. Il est essentiel de les repérer afin de bien comprendre l'enchaînement des idées et la structure d'un texte. Voici une liste des principaux mots de liaison qui traduisent entre autres :

• La cause

as *(comme)*, **because** *(parce que)*, **because of** *(à cause de)*, **for** *(car)*, **since** *(puisque)*, **thanks to** *(grâce à)*...
Exemple : As a medical student you have to do a placement in this hospital.

• L'addition

indeed *(en effet, en outre)*, **besides** *(par ailleurs)*, **moreover** *(en outre, de plus)*...
Exemple : He didn't want to go out. Besides, he was too tired.

• La conséquence

consequently *(par conséquent)*, **so** *(alors)*, **therefore** *(donc, par conséquent)*, **thus** *(ainsi)*, **hence** *(d'où)*,...
Exemple : She didn't work for the exam. Consequently, she failed.

• La restriction

despite *(malgré)*, **in spite of** *(en dépit de)*, **unless** *(à moins que)* ...
Exemple : Despite his efforts, he didn't convince me.

• La condition

if *(si)*, **provided** *(à condition que)*, **even if** *(même si)*, **unless** *(à moins que)*, **since** *(puisque)*...
Exemple : He can eat, provided that you help him.

• L'opposition

although/though *(bien que)*, **but** *(mais)*, **however** *(cependant)*, **whereas, while** *(alors que, tandis que)*, **yet** *(pourtant)*, **nevertheless** *(néanmoins)*...
Exemple : Although/though she was thirsty, she didn't drink anything.

• Le temps

when *(quand, lorsque)*, **while** *(pendant que)*, **as** *(tandis que, comme)*, **till, until** *(jusqu'à ce que)*, **as soon as** *(dès que)*, **as long as** *(tant que)*, **since** *(depuis que)*...
Exemple : We waited until 9:30, but she didn't come.

• Le but

in order to *(pour, en vue de)*, **so that** *(afin que, de sorte que)*...
Exemple : I talked to her very quietly, so that she wouldn't feel left out.

• L'exemple

for example, for instance, e.g *(par exemple)*, **such as** *(tel que)*...
Exemple : For example, if you fast, you may purify your body and your mind.

Exercice 1

Réponse p. 200

Associez le mot de liaison avec son équivalent français.

1. In spite of .... •		• .... A. Tandis que, comme
2. Whereas .... •		• .... B. Si
3. If .... •		• .... C. Alors que, tandis que
4. As .... •		• .... D. En dépit de
5. Unless .... •		• .... E. Par conséquent
6. Provided .... •		• .... F. À cause de
7. Because of .... •		• .... G. À condition que
8. Consequently .... •		• .... H. À moins que
9. Since .... •		• .... I. Même si
10. So that .... •		• .... J. Jusqu'à ce que
11. Even if .... •		• .... K. Afin que, de sorte que
12. Until .... •		• .... L. Depuis que, Puisque
13. While .... •		• .... M. Grâce à
14. As long as .... •		• .... N. Bien que
15. Although, though .... •		• .... O. Tant que
16. Thanks to .... •		• .... P. Pendant que

Exercice 2

Réponse p. 200

Soulignez les mots de liaison et traduisez les phrases.

1. If someone in your family has died from cancer, you should have regular check-ups.

....

2. Some cancers develop slowly whereas others spread much faster.

....

3. Thanks to an early diagnosis, many cancers can be treated successfully.

....

4. Don't hesitate to report any unusual symptoms such as a lump or a mole that changes colour.

....

Exercice 3 : Palliative care team in hospitals, at home and home for dependant elderly people*

Réponse p. 200

In the palliative care team, nurses have a fundamental role. The palliative care team puts the patients and their families at the centre of all decisions. They take a patient's physical, psychological, mental, spiritual, social and practical aspects into account*.

Associez les professions à leur équivalent en anglais et écrivez-les dans l'organigramme ci-dessous.

1. Aide-soignant(e) .... •	• .... **A.** Nurse
2. Bénévole .... •	• .... **B.** Healthcare assistant
3. Médecin .... •	• .... **C.** Social worker
4. Psychologue .... •	• .... **D.** Homecare assistant
5. Infirmier(ère) .... •	• .... **E.** Volunteer
6. Kinésithérapeute .... •	• .... **F.** Physician/Doctor
7. Auxiliaire de vie .... •	• .... **G.** Physiotherapist
8. Travailleur social .... •	• .... **H.** Psychologist
9. Aumônier .... •	• .... **I.** Chaplain

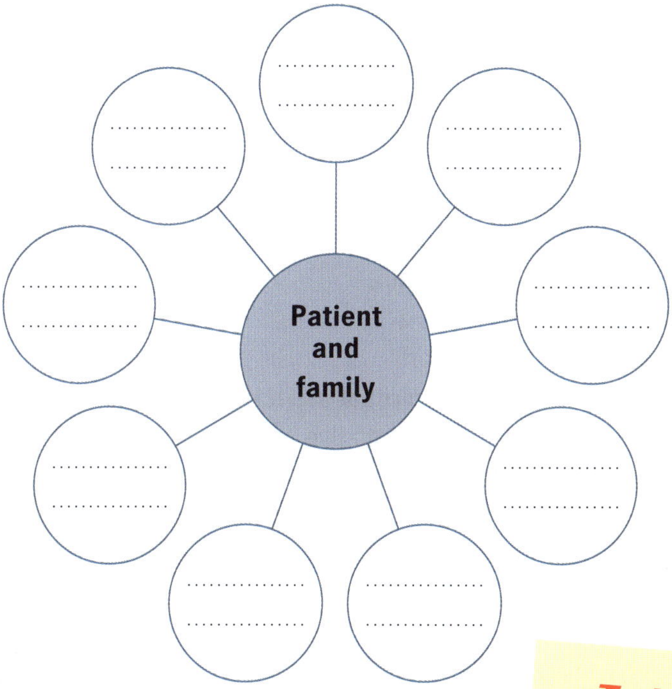

To help you

- **Hole for dependant elderly people:** EHPAD
- **To take into account:** prendre en compte

Exercice 4 : The palliative approach

Réponse p. 201

Après avoir lu le texte, rayez les principes contraires à ceux d'un service de soins palliatifs et remplacez-les par les mots corrects.

The palliative approach uses palliative care principles, for example: dignity, hope, discomfort*, quality of life, relief of suffering. These principles are used with people facing chronic, life-limiting conditions* at all stages, not just at the end of life. Attitudes and principles for successful palliative care involve empathy and compassion, insensitivity and demonstrate anxiety for the patient.

> **To help you**
> - **discomfort:** gêne
> - **condition:** état

....

....

....

....

....

....

....

Exercice 5 : The 5 principles of palliative care

Réponse p. 201

Complétez les phrases ci-dessous avec les mots de l'encadré.

• actively	• death	• patient care
• normal process	• relief	

Palliative care

1. It provides .... from pain.
2. It affirms life and considers dying as a ....
3. It intends neither to hasten* or put off* ....
4. It integrates the psychological and spiritual aspects of ....
5. It offers a support system to help patients live as .... as possible until death.

> **To help you**
> - **to hasten:** accélérer, hâter
> - **to put off:** remettre à plus tard, repousser

Exercice 6 : End-of-life situation

Réponse p. 201

Après avoir lu les quatre phrases ci-dessous, cochez la bonne réponse dans le tableau.

- In England, most people want to die at home, but only 20 - 30% do so. About 55% of the population ends up dying in a hospital.
- Patients with chronic illnesses or disabilities may need palliative care.
- The main goal of end-of-life care is to relieve physical and mental suffering.
- In an end-of-life situation nurses have to provide care for the dying patient and care for the patient's family.

	True	False
1. In England, most people die at home by their own choice.		
2. A patient admitted to a Nursing Care Facility for management of Alzheimer's disease is a good example of palliative care.		
3. End-of-life suffering can be prevented if physical pain is medicated.		
4. Nursing care* for the dying patient also includes considering some of the patient's family needs		

Exercice 7 : Options available to people looking for palliative care

Réponse p. 201

Associez chaque élément de la première colonne à son équivalent français.

1. Palliative care in hospitals..... •
2. Palliative nursing in a care home....................................... •
3. Day care at a hospice palliative care*......................... •
4. Palliative home care............... •
5. Care in a care facility............. •

- • .... **A.** Soins palliatifs à domicile
- • .... **B.** Soins palliatifs dans une maison de santé
- • .... **C.** Soins dans un établissement de soins
- • .... **D.** Soins palliatifs à l'hôpital
- • .... **E.** Soins de jour dans un établissement de soins palliatifs

To help you

- **nursing care:** soins infirmiers
- **hospice palliative care:** établissement de soins palliatifs

Dialogue between Mr Fear and the nurse

Traduction p. 219

A nurse is answering Mr Fear's questions about his father's condition

Mr Fear Good afternoon. I think my father is sleeping a lot lately*. Is it due to the morphine?

Nurse Yes. The treatment he is given and the development of his illness tend* to make him sleep. This clinical manifestation is the result of a slowdown* in his body's functions*. We try to reduce his pain so that he doesn't get exhausted from fighting* it.

Mr Fear And could you explain to me why you are giving him all these treatments?

Nurse You know, without them, his life would be unbearable*. He could swallow his medication until now, but he can't do it any longer. This is why we have to give them intravenously. The doctor has not changed the morphine dosage and he has given him a tranquilliser* to make him calmer and more relaxed*.

Mr Fear All right.

Nurse Tell me, Mr Fear when you last met the doctor, did he tell you why your father was transferred to palliative care?

Mr Fear Yes, he did. He told me he was a specialist in pain care and explained to me what palliative care is. I've understood that your goal is not to cure but to improve my father's quality of life and relieve his symptoms.

Nurse That's it. You have understood the essential thing.

Mr Fear I met the oncologist too who explained to me the development of his illness but I didn't think my father was at the end of his life.

Nurse As you can see he has difficulty breathing, oedema and noisy breathing. These are common symptoms at the end of life.

Mr Fear Do you mean he may die at any time?

Nurse Yes, he may, even if it is impossible to know when it will happen precisely.

Mr Fear Thank you very much for all* you are doing for him and me. May I stay with him tonight?

Nurse Certainly, we'll bring an extra bed for you. You know, you can talk to him to reassure him, even if your father doesn't seem to react to your words he can probably hear you.

To help you

- **lately:** ces derniers jours, récemment
- **to tend to:** avoir tendance à
- **slowdown:** ralentissement
- **body functions:** organisme
- **to fight:** lutter
- **unbearable:** insupportable
- **tranquiliser:** anxiolytique
- **relaxed:** détendu
- **for all:** tout ce que

Questions sur le dialogue

1. Why is Mr Fear's father sleeping a lot recently? ....

....

....

2. Why is Mr Fear's father given all these treatments? ....

....

....

3. How does the nurse know Mr Fear's father is at the end of his life? ....

....

....

Travaillez à deux : Common symptoms at the end of life or physical signs of impending* death.

Réponse p. 201

A. asks B.: Which are the two symptoms that do not correspond to the common symptoms at the end of life?

	Yes	No
Delirium		
Shortness of breath		
Coughing		
Eczema		
Constipation		
Trouble swallowing		

B. asks A.: Which are the two symptoms that do not correspond to the common symptoms at the end of life?

	Yes	No
Loss of appetite		
Difficulty breathing		
Urticaria (hives)		
Changes in urination		
Swelling* to feet, ankles and hands		
Increased* physical weakness		
Diabetes		

To help you

- **impending:** imminent
- **swelling:** gonflement
- **increased:** accru

Exercice 8 : Communication with dying patients

Réponse p. 201

Complétez les textes avec les mots de l'encadré.

- misunderstanding*
- considered
- distress
- bereavement*
- end of life care

Good communication with a dying person improves his or her .... and the .... experience. It can help to ensure that the dying person's wishes are .... Good communication avoids .... and unnecessary.. .

- encouraging questions
- sensitive way
- carefully
- to talk about death
- an honest
- being ready

These following points have a great effect on dying patients:

- talking with them in .... way;
- .... to talk about dying;
- giving bad news in a .... ;
- listening .... to them;
- .... from them;
- being sensitive when they are ready ....

To help you

- **misunderstanding:** incompréhension
- **bereavement:** perte, deuil

Exercice 9

Réponse p. 202

Écrivez dans le tableau le groupe de mots correspondant à sa définition et son équivalent en français.

- Advance health directive
- A support person or a trusted person
- Living will
- Therapeutic obstinacy

Group of words	Translation into French	Definitions
		A legal document in which a person specifies what actions should be taken for their health if they are no longer able to make decisions for themselves because of illness or incapacity.
		A person who gives support to a patient and makes medical decisions in his or her interest when they lose the capacity to express themselves.
		It is the oldest form of advance directive leaving instructions for treatment.
		The use of aggressive treatment to prolong the life of a patient in the terminal stages of an illness with no real hope of improving her or his condition.

Exercice 10 : Providing emotional comfort to the patient

Réponse p. 202

Some emotions are common to most dying patients. These emotions include fear of abandonment and fear of being a burden*. Patients are also concerned by* loss* of dignity and loss of control.

Palliative-care nurses not only manage pain and other symptoms but they assist patients in the process of death with dignity. They can provide comfort by:

- keeping the patient company by talking, reading, or just being with him or her;
- allowing the person to express fears and concerns about dying;
- being willing to hear about the person's life;
- avoiding refusing to give difficult information. Most patients prefer to be included in* discussions about issues* that concern them;
- reassuring the patient that you will honour his or her advance directives;
- asking if there is anything you can do;
- respecting the patient's need for privacy.

To help you

- **burden:** poids
- **to be concerned by:** s'inquiéter de, être inquiet de
- **loss:** perte
- **to be included in:** participer
- **issue:** problème, question, point

Associez chaque verbe à son équivalent français.

1. Keep company .... •
2. Allow .... •
3. Be willing to .... •
4. Avoid .... •
5. Reassure .... •
6. Ask .... •
7. Respect .... •

• .... **A.** Respecter
• .... **B.** Demander
• .... **C.** Rassurer
• .... **D.** Tenir compagnie
• .... **E.** Permettre
• .... **F.** Être prêt, disposé
• .... **G.** Éviter

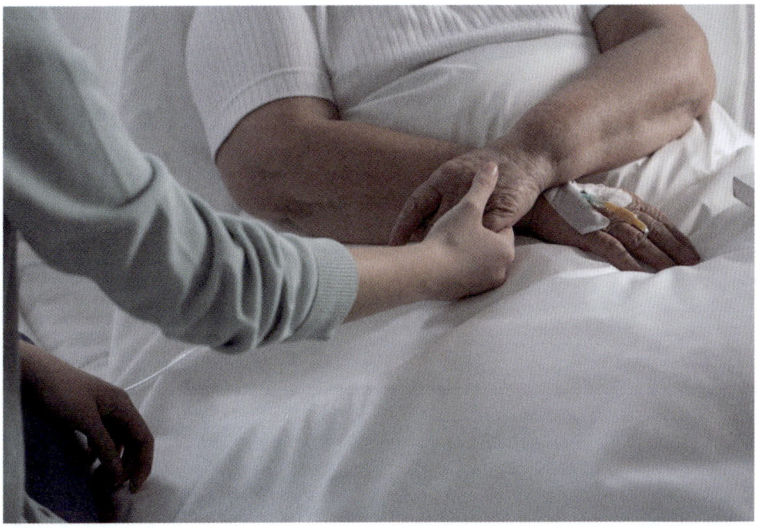

Condolences or sympathies

What you should say to someone who is mourning the loss* of a loved one*:

- I'm deeply saddened by the loss of your daughter;
- Please accept my condolences and do not hesitate to contact me, especially during this difficult time;
- Our sincere sympathies to you and your family;
- My deepest sympathies* go to you and your family;
- Please accept my condolences on the passing* of your husband. It was an honour to have known such a great person and I will truly miss him*;
- May her/his soul* rest in peace.

To help you

- **to mourn the loss:** vivre le deuil
- **a loved one:** un être cher
- **deepest sympathies:** sincères condoléances
- **passing:** mort
- **I will truly miss him:** il me manquera beaucoup
- **soul:** âme

Si vous deviez rédiger une carte de condoléances, choisissez parmi les expressions ci-dessus celle qui vous conviendrait le mieux, puis écrivez-la sur la carte.

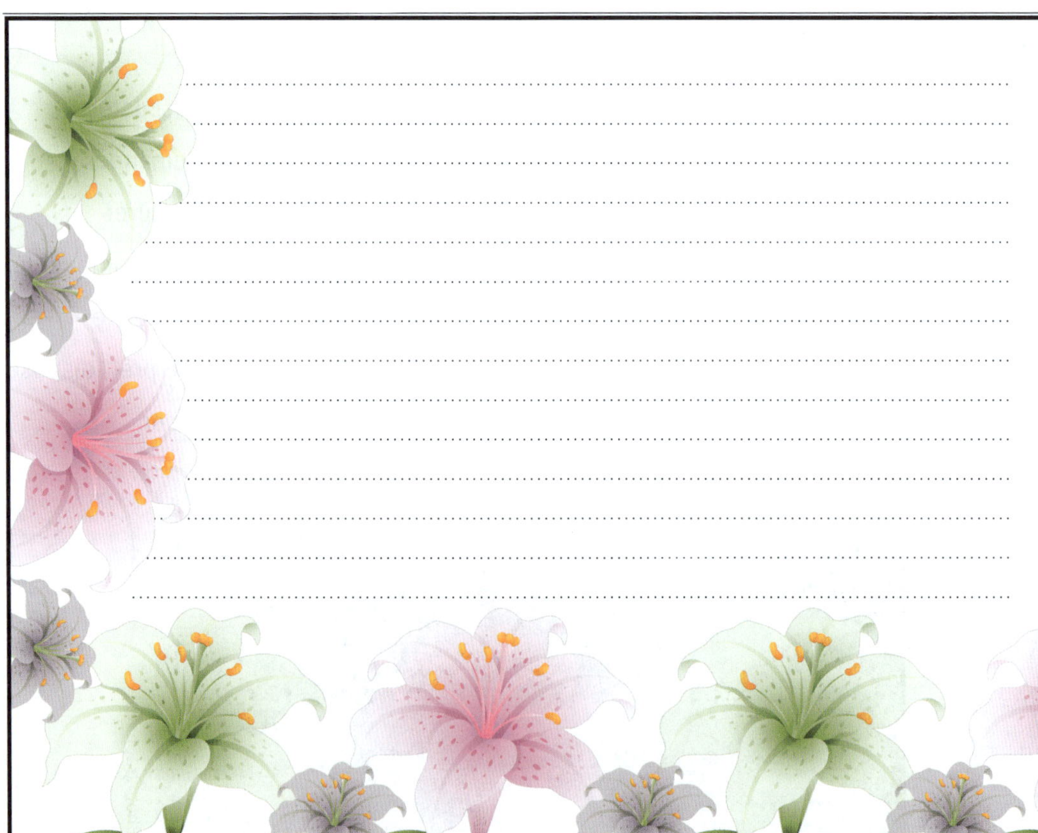

Exercice 11 : Repatriation

Traduction p. 220
Réponse p. 202

Complétez la conversation entre l'infirmière et Mme Brown à l'aide des phrases suivantes :

- … your husband had a pacemaker.
- … deepest sympathy …
- … the funeral directors*…
- … choose a coffin*.
- … to repatriate my husband's body
- … to the mortuary…

A nurse is giving information to Mrs Brown about administrative, repatriation procedures and funeral arrangements for her husband's body.

Nurse First of all, my **(1)** .... to you, Mrs Brown.

Mrs Brown Thank you very much. Could you tell me what I have to do **(2)** .... to Ireland?

Nurse Certainly. First of all, you have to notify* the town hall of his death.

Mrs Brown All right. Do I have to do it today?

Nurse Not necessarily. In fact, you have forty-eight hours. Don't forget to take the death certificate.

Mrs Brown Have you got a listing of **(3)** ...., please?

Nurse Yes. Here it is. You can call them this morning. They will help you to **(4)** ....

Mrs Brown Do I have to contact the airline?

Nurse No, it isn't necessary. The funeral directors will arrange the flight. You must show them your husband's passport or ID* and give them your telephone number and the name and address of the funeral directors in Ireland.

Mrs Brown How many days will it take?

Nurse I don't know exactly. A few days, I suppose. It depends on the flights.

Mrs Brown In the meantime* what happens?

Nurse The body will be transferred **(5)** .... where it will remain* until it is put it in the coffin*.

Mrs Brown And what about a cremation?

Nurse You again have to contact the funeral directors. But don't forget to tell them **(6)** .... They have to remove* it before the cremation.

Mrs Brown Thank you very much for your help.

Nurse Not at all.

To help you

- **to notify:** déclarer
- **funeral directors:** pompes funèbres
- **coffin:** cercueil
- **ID:** carte d'identité *(identity card)*
- **In the meantime:** en attendant
- **to remain:** rester
- **to put (it) in the coffin:** mettre en bière
- **to remove:** enlever

http://www.lienmini.fr/angsoinq13a

Vocabulary quiz

Réponse p. 202

Complétez chaque affirmation avec le bon terme.

1. In the palliative care .... nurses have a fundamental role.

a) aspect **b)** team **c)** point of view **d)** distress

2. Nurses .... patient's physical and psychological aspects .... account.

a) take .... in **b)** take .... out **c)** take .... into **d)** take .... off

3. The palliative approach uses care principles such as dignity, hope and.........

a) discomfort* **b)** happyness **c)** need **d)** quality

4. The nurse offers a support system to help patients live as .... as possible until death.

a) quickly **b)** slowly **c)** actively **d)** passively

5. End-of-life suffering can be .... if physical pain is medicated.

a) given **b)** influenced **c)** considered **d)** prevented

http://www.lienmini.fr/angsoinq13b

Vocabulary quiz

Réponse p. 202

Complétez chaque affirmation avec le bon terme.

1. Some emotions are common to most dying patients, they include fear of being a ....

a) pain **b)** relief **c)** burden* **d)** problem

2. Advance .... is a legal document in which a person specifies which actions should be taken for their health because of their incapacity to make decision.

a) will **b)** directive **c)** file **d)** case

3. A nurse can keep .... by talking, reading or just being with the patient.

a) reassurance **b)** assistance **c)** help **d)** company

4. The family has 48 hours to bring the death .... to the town hall.

a) document **b)** certificate **c)** directive **d)** file

5. The body is transferred to the morgue where it will remain until the funeral .... put it in the coffin.

a) head **b)** manager **c)** directors **d)** employee

To help you

- **discomfort:** gêne, inconfort, malaise
- **burden:** poids

Medical Vocabulary: unit 13

- **life-threatening:** extrêmement grave
- **life expectancy:** espérance de vie
- **hospice:** établissement de soins palliatifs
- **bereavement:** perte, deuil
- **loss:** perte
- **funeral directors:** pompes funèbres
- **advance health directive:** directives anticipées
- **a trusted person / support person:** personne de confiance
- **therapeutic obstinacy:** obstination déraisonnable/acharnement thérapeutique

Let's discuss!

What is palliative care at home?

Corrigés

Exercice 1

1. In spite of	A. Tandis que, comme
2. Whereas	B. Si
3. If	C. Alors que, tandis que
4. As	D. En dépit de
5. Unless	E. Par conséquent
6. Provided	F. À cause de
7. Because of	G. À condition que
8. Consequently	H. À moins que
9. Since	I. Même si
10. So that	J. Jusqu'à ce que
11. Even if	K. Afin que, de sorte que
12. Until	L. Depuis que, puisque
13. While	M. Grâce à
14. As long as	N. Bien que
15. Although, though	O. Tant que
16. Thanks to	P. Pendant que

Exercice 2

1. **If** someone in your family has died from cancer, you should have regular check-ups.
Si quelqu'un dans votre famille est mort d'un cancer, vous devez (devriez) être surveillé régulièrement.

2. Some cancers develop slowly **whereas** others spread much faster.
Certains cancers évoluent lentement, alors que d'autres progressent bien plus rapidement.

3. **Thanks to** an early diagnosis, many cancers can be treated successfully.
Grâce à un diagnostic précoce, de nombreux cancers peuvent être traités avec succès.

4. Don't hesitate to report any unusual symptoms **such as** a lump or a mole that changes colour.
N'hésitez pas à signaler tout symptôme inhabituel, tel qu'une grosseur ou un grain de beauté qui change de couleur.

Exercice 3

1. Aide-soignant(e)	A. Nurse
2. Bénévole	B. Healthcare assistant
3. Médecin	C. Social worker
4. Psychologue	D. Homecare assistant
5. Infirmier(ère)	E. Volunteer
6. Kinésithérapeute	F. Physician/Doctor
7. Auxiliaire de vie	G. Physiotherapist
8. Travailleur social	H. Psychologist
9. Aumônier	I. Chaplain

Exercice 4

The palliative approach uses palliative care principles, for example: dignity, hope, ~~discomfort~~ **comfort**, quality of life, relief of suffering. These principles are used with people facing chronic, life-limiting conditions at all stages, not just at the end of life. Attitudes and principles for successful palliative care involve empathy and compassion, ~~insensitivity~~ **sensitivity** and demonstrate ~~anxiety~~ **concern** for the patient.

Exercice 5

1. It provides **relief** from pain.
2. It affirms life and considers dying as a **normal process**.
3. It intends neither to hasten* or put off* **death**.
4. It integrates the psychological and spiritual aspects of **patient care**.
5. It offers a support system to help patients live as **actively** as possible until death.

Exercice 6

1. False 2. True 3. False 4. True

Exercice 7

1. Palliative care in hospitals.
2. Palliative nursing in a care home
3. Day care at a hospice palliative care
4. Palliative home care
5. Care in a care facility

A. Soins palliatifs à domicile
B. Soins palliatifs dans une maison de santé
C. Soins dans un établissement de soins
D. Soins palliatifs à l'hôpital
E. Soins de jour dans un établissement de soins palliatifs

Travaillez à deux

	Yes	No
Delirium	✖	
Shortness of breath	✖	
Coughing	✖	
Miningitis		✖
Eczema		✖
Constipation	✖	
Trouble swallowing	✖	

	Yes	No
Loss of appetite	✖	
Difficulty breathing	✖	
Urticaria (hives)		✖
Changes in urination	✖	
Swelling* to feet, ankles and hands	✖	
Increased* physical weakness	✖	
Diabetes		✖

Exercice 8

Good communication with a dying person improves their **end of life care** and the **bereavement** experience of those important to them. It can help to ensure that the dying person's wishes are **considered.** Good communication avoids **misunderstanding** and unnecessary **distress**.

These following points have a great effect on dying patients:
- talking with them in an honest way;
- being ready to talk about dying;
- giving bad news in a sensitive way;
- listening carefully to them;
- encouraging questions from them;
- being sensitive when they are ready to talk about death.

Exercice 9

Group of words	Translation into French	Definitions
Advance health directive	Directives anticipées	A legal document in which a person specifies what actions should be taken for their health if they are no longer able to make decisions for themselves because of illness or incapacity
A trusted person or a support person	Personne de confiance	A person who gives support to a patient and makes medical decisions in his or her interest when they lose the capacity to express themselves
Living will	Testament de vie	It is the oldest form of advance directive leaving instructions for treatment
Therapeutic obstinacy	Obstination déraisonnable ou acharnement thérapeutique	The use of aggressive treatment to prolong the life of a patient in the terminal stages of an illness with no real hope of improving her or his condition

Exercice 10

1. Keep company
2. Allow
3. Be willing to
4. Avoid
5. Reassure
6. Ask
7. Respect

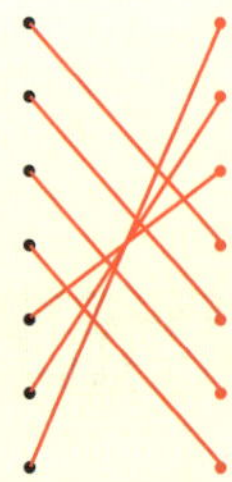

A. Respecter
B. Demander
C. Rassurer
D. Tenir compagnie
E. Permettre
F. Être prêt, disposé
G. Éviter

Exercice 11

1. … deepest sympathy…
2. … to repatriate my husband's body…
3. … the funeral directors, …
4. … choose a coffin.
5. … to the mortuary…
6. … your husband had a pacemaker.

Vocabulary quiz

1. team 2. take… into 3. discomfort 4. actively 5. prevented

Vocabulary quiz

1. burden 2. directive 3. company 4. certificate 5. directors

Traduction des dialogues

Unit 1

Piste 1 Accueillir un patient aux urgences

Voir p. 2

M. Brown est admis à l'hôpital.

M. Brown	Bonjour. Je me suis blessé. Pouvez-vous m'aider, s'il vous plaît ?
Infirmière	Bien sûr. Parlez-vous français ?
M. Brown	Non, pas du tout. Je suis désolé.
Infirmière	Que s'est-il passé ?
M. Brown	Je suis tombé d'une échelle.
Infirmière	Où avez-vous mal ?
M. Brown	J'ai mal à la jambe. Je pense qu'elle est cassée.
Infirmière	*(S'adressant à une autre infirmière)* Pouvez-vous amener une attelle gonflable, s'il vous plaît ? *(S'adressant à M. Brown)* Ne vous inquiétez pas. Tout va bien se passer. Pouvez-vous vous allonger sur le brancard ?

Au box des urgences.

Infirmière	Êtes-vous allergique à des médicaments, l'aspirine par exemple ?
M. Brown	Non, mais je suis allergique à l'iode et à la pénicilline.
Infirmière	Je vais vous donner un antalgique par voie intraveineuse. Vous êtes relié au moniteur afin que je puisse lire votre rythme cardiaque.
M. Brown	Je prends un médicament pour l'hypertension artérielle.
Infirmière	Prenez-vous d'autres médicaments ?
M. Brown	Oui, mais je ne me souviens pas de leurs noms. Je suis diabétique et je fais de l'angine de poitrine.
Infirmière	Avez-vous déjà été opéré ?
M. Brown	Oui, il y a cinq ans pour la vésicule biliaire.
Infirmière	Fumez-vous ?
M. Brown	Oui, je fume à peu près vingt cigarettes par jour.

Piste 2 Remplir une fiche d'admission

Voir p. 7

Réceptionniste	Excusez-moi. Pourriez-vous me donner des renseignements concernant votre mari, s'il vous plaît ? J'ai besoin de remplir une fiche d'admission. Quel est son nom de famille, s'il vous plaît ?
Mme Brown	Brown.
Réceptionniste	Pourriez-vous l'épeler ?
Mme Brown	B.R.O.W.N.
Réceptionniste	Quel est son prénom ?
Mme Brown	James.
Réceptionniste	Où est-il né ?

Mme Brown	À Bath, en Angleterre.
Réceptionniste	Maintenant j'ai besoin de renseignements complémentaires concernant votre adresse. Où habitez-vous en ce moment ?
Mme Brown	Nous habitons à Ruffec, 21, rue Aunay.
Réceptionniste	Quelle est votre adresse personnelle ?
Mme Brown	12, Raven Street, à Bath, en Angleterre.
Réceptionniste	Pourriez-vous parler plus lentement, s'il vous plaît ? Merci. Quel est votre numéro de téléphone en France ?
Mme Brown	05 45 12 43 76.
Réceptionniste	Avez-vous une couverture sociale ? Bien pourriez-vous me donner votre carte mutuelle et votre carte européenne, s'il vous plaît ?
Mme Brown	Oui. Les voici.
Réceptionniste	Merci. Quel est le nom de votre médecin traitant ?
Mme Brown	Dr Daniels, 12, London Street, à Bath.

Unit 2

Piste 7

Demander son chemin

Voir p. 18

Le fils de M. Brown, Mike, est sur le chemin de l'hôpital pour rendre visite à son père.

Mike	Excusez-moi. Pourriez-vous m'indiquer le chemin pour aller à l'hôpital, s'il vous plaît ?
Dame	Bien sûr. C'est à l'angle de la rue principale. Allez tout droit, puis tournez à droite avant le rond-point.
Mike	Est-ce après les feux ?
Dame	Oui, en face de la pharmacie, à côté de la poste.
Mike	À quelle distance est-ce précisément ?
Dame	À peu près dix minutes à pied.
Mike	Merci beaucoup.
Dame	De rien.

Quelques minutes plus tard, à l'accueil de l'hôpital.

Mike	Je voudrais rendre visite à M. Brown. Pourriez-vous m'indiquer où est sa chambre ?
Réceptionniste	Oui, il est dans le service de médecine.
Mike	C'est à quel étage ?
Réceptionniste	C'est au troisième étage.
Mike	Y a-t-il un ascenseur ?
Réceptionniste	Oui, au bout du couloir. Prenez l'ascenseur jusqu'au troisième. Quand vous sortez, tournez à gauche, puis suivez le couloir. C'est la troisième porte sur votre gauche.
Mike	Merci.
Réceptionniste	Je vous en prie.

Piste 9 Un appel téléphonique

Voir p. 23

Réceptionniste	Bonjour, service de médecine. Puis-je vous aider ?
Demandeur	Puis-je parler au chef de service ou au cadre de santé qui s'occupe de M. Newton, s'il vous plaît ?
Réceptionniste	C'est de la part de qui ?
Demandeur	Dr Roberts à l'appareil.
Réceptionniste	Je suis désolée, mais il est absent aujourd'hui et le cadre de santé est en réunion. Je vous passe une de ses secrétaires. Ne quittez pas, s'il vous plaît… Je suis vraiment désolée, la ligne est occupée.
Demandeur	Puis-je laisser un message ?
Réceptionniste	Oui, bien sûr.
Demandeur	Pourriez vous lui dire de me rappeler aussi vite que possible ?
Réceptionniste	Pourriez-vous me redonner votre nom, s'il vous plaît ?
Demandeur	Dr Roberts de Paris et mon numéro de téléphone est le 01 47 58 58 99.
Réceptionniste	Très bien. Dr Roberts. Je transmettrai votre message.
Demandeur	Au revoir.
Réceptionniste	Au revoir.

Unit 3

Piste 11 Faire un pansement

Voir p. 34

Le dialogue se passe entre un infirmier et une élève infirmière. M. Brown a été opéré il y a deux jours pour réduire sa fracture ; il est en chirurgie orthopédique. Le chirurgien a coupé une fenêtre dans son plâtre pour faire le pansement. La plaie de M. Brown est purulente. On change ses pansements deux fois par jour. Maud, une étudiante en soins infirmiers, s'entretient avec l'infirmier de M. Brown. Elle va changer son pansement.

Infirmier	Maud, commençons ensemble la procédure, puis vous pourrez changer le pansement de M. Brown. Bien, par quoi commencez-vous ?
Étudiante	D'abord je me présente au patient, puis je mets mes gants pour empêcher des microbes de pénétrer dans la plaie.
Infirmier	Pourquoi ?
Étudiante	Parce que ça pourrait causer une infection. Ensuite, je nettoie la plaie avec un antiseptique et j'applique une compresse stérile.
Infirmier	Et à quoi sert le drain ?
Étudiante	À enlever le pus.
Infirmier	Bien. Et que se passe-t-il en cas d'infection ?
Étudiante	Eh bien, nous prélevons un échantillon avec un coton-tige stérile et nous l'envoyons aux laboratoires.
Infirmier	C'est ça. Quand retirez-vous le drain ?

Étudiante	Je le retirerai petit à petit, lorsque la plaie ne sera plus purulente. Si c'est le cas, je demanderai d'abord au chirurgien de venir voir.
Infirmier	Et les agrafes de M. Brown ? Excusez-moi, ses points?
Étudiante	J'enlèverai les points dans deux ou trois jours.
Infirmier	Qu'est-ce que vous utilisez pour les enlever ?
Étudiante	Ça dépend. Un coupe-fil, des ciseaux, ou on peut utiliser un scalpel ou une lame.
Infirmier	Bien. Alors Maud, êtes-vous prête à changer le pansement de M. Brown ?
Étudiante	Tout à fait.
Infirmier	Je reste avec vous au cas où vous auriez besoin de moi.

Un peu plus tard avec M. Brown.

Infirmier	Est-ce que votre femme vient aujourd'hui, M. Brown ?
M. Brown	Oui, elle vient cet après-midi. Elle s'inquiète beaucoup, vous savez. Pourriez-vous lui remonter un peu le moral ? Elle est tellement anxieuse.
Infirmier	Bien sûr, je lui parlerai quand elle arrivera.

Piste 12

Élimination urinaire

Voir p. 39

Infirmier	Vous avez besoin de quelque chose ?
Patiente (mal à l'aise)	J'aimerais faire… euh… faire…
Infirmier	Je suis désolé mais je ne comprends pas.
Patiente	J'aimerais faire pipi.
Infirmier	Oh, excusez-moi, vous voulez dire que vous avez besoin d'aller aux toilettes.
Patiente	Oui, exactement.
Infirmier	Je vous mets le bassin. Voici du papier toilette. Appelez-moi avec cette sonnette quand vous aurez fini.
Patiente	Merci.
Infirmier	Je vous en prie.

Quelques minutes plus tard.

Infirmier	Vos urines sont troubles. Je vais donc envoyer un échantillon au laboratoire. Avez-vous des problèmes quand vous urinez ?
Patiente	Pas vraiment, mais ça brûle un peu.

Le jour suivant.

Infirmier	Le médecin veut que vous ayez une sonde urinaire. Ne vous inquiétez pas. Je vais vous poser la sonde et l'insérer tout doucement dans votre vessie, puis je vais vous mettre une poche pour récupérer vos urines.

Unit 4

Piste 15 Obtenir des renseignements concernant les antécédents

Voir p. 48

Hier, M. Brown a présenté des complications cardiaques. Le Dr Lavau pose des questions à Mme Brown concernant l'histoire personnelle de son mari. Il veut savoir si, dans sa famille, il y a eu des antécédents particuliers.

Dr Lavau Savez-vous s'il y a des problèmes d'hypertension artérielle dans sa famille ?

Mme Brown Non, je ne pense pas.

Dr Lavau Y a-t-il des cas de crises cardiaques ou d'attaques ?

Mme Brown Une fois, il m'a dit que son grand-père du côté de sa mère était mort subitement d'une crise cardiaque. En ce qui concerne ses parents, son père est mort, il y a trois ans.

Dr Lavau De quoi est-il mort ?

Mme Brown Il est mort d'un cancer des poumons.

Dr Lavau Votre mari est-il un gros fumeur ?

Mme Brown Oh, oui. Il fume au moins 25 cigarettes par jour.

Dr Lavau Hier, j'ai vu sur son dossier médical qu'il fait de l'angine de poitrine. Fait-il du sport ou a-t-il une activité physique régulière ?

Mme Brown Il jardine beaucoup, c'est tout.

Dr Lavau Avant hier, a-t-il déjà eu des douleurs de poitrine ?

Mme Brown Oui, mais il pensait que ce n'était rien de sérieux alors que je lui ai dit que ça pouvait l'être. J'ai remarqué, il y a quelques mois, qu'il avait des essoufflements.

Dr Lavau Merci beaucoup, Mme Brown.

Piste 17 La douleur

Voir p. 53

Infirmière Comment allez-vous aujourd'hui ?

Patient Je ne me sens pas très bien. Mon genou me fait mal.

Infirmière Que ressentez-vous comme douleur ?

Patient C'est difficile à dire.

Infirmière Est-ce une douleur aiguë ou légère ?

Patient Je ne peux pas dire précisément. C'est une douleur constante.

Infirmière Pourriez-vous me montrer où vous avez mal ?

Patient Ici, exactement.

Infirmière Si la douleur continue, je demanderai au docteur si je peux vous donner un calmant pour vous soulager.

Patient J'ai également un léger mal de tête. Je me sens tellement fatigué aujourd'hui.

Infirmière C'est tout à fait normal, vous savez. Vous avez été opéré hier. Ne vous inquiétez pas, vous souffrirez moins demain.

Unit 5

Piste 20

Examen clinique et *nursing*

Voir p. 64

Le Dr Martin examine M. Brown à cause de ses complications cardiaques. Elle lui explique ce qu'elle est en train de faire.

Dr Martin	Tout d'abord, je vais vérifier votre cœur. Pourriez-vous vous asseoir ?
M. Brown	Bien sûr.
Dr Martin	Pourriez-vous enlever le haut de votre pyjama ? Merci. Ouvrez la bouche et respirez profondément. Je veux écouter votre respiration. Je suis désolée, le stéthoscope est froid, n'est-ce pas ?
M. Brown	Oh, oui.
Dr Martin	Inspirez, puis expirez la bouche ouverte. Doucement, s'il vous plaît. Maintenant toussez. C'est bien. Retenez votre respiration. Est-ce que ça vous fait mal quand j'appuie ici ?
M. Brown	Un peu.
Dr Martin	Bien, vous pouvez vous rhabiller, M. Brown. Merci beaucoup.

Quelques minutes plus tard, une aide-soignante vient faire la toilette de M. Brown au lit.

Aide-soignante	C'est l'heure de vous laver, M. Brown. L'eau, ça va ?
M. Brown	Oui. J'aimerais me raser aujourd'hui.
Aide-soignante	Bien sûr. Où sont votre crème à raser et votre rasoir ?
M. Brown	Dans mon placard.
Aide-soignante	Demain, vous vous laverez dans la salle de bain.
M. Brown	Formidable ! Je prendrai une douche et je me laverai les cheveux.
Aide-soignante	Pourriez-vous lever votre bras ? Merci. Pourriez-vous vous tourner ? J'applique de la pommade sur vos fesses. Est-ce que ça va ? C'est pour éviter les escarres.
M. Brown	Pourriez-vous mettre mon pyjama dans ce sac ? Ma femme le ramènera à la maison pour le laver.

Piste 22

Conseiller une patiente qui a un plâtre

Voir p. 69

Médecin	J'ai dû réduire votre fracture avant de vous poser votre plâtre.
Patiente	« Réduire » ? Qu'est-ce que cela veut dire docteur ?
Médecin	On a remis en place les deux parties de votre péroné.
Patiente	Oh, je vois.
Médecin	Le plâtre est-il trop serré ?
Patiente	Non, ça va.
Médecin	Avant de quitter l'hôpital, je dois vous donner quelques conseils. Il faut 48 heures à un plâtre pour sécher. Aussi, vous devez le garder au sec.
Patiente	Bien sûr. Je peux marcher ?

Médecin	Vous pouvez marcher avec des cannes anglaises. Mais informez-moi immédiatement si vous ressentez une perte de sensibilité ou si votre pied devient froid.
Patiente	D'accord, c'est entendu.
Médecin	Je dois vous donner un conseil supplémentaire. Vous devez me prévenir immédiatement si vous sentez une odeur anormale.

Unit 6

Piste 25 Faire une prise de sang et changer une perfusion

Voir p. 78

Après son opération, M. Brown a fait des complications cardiaques : une embolie pulmonaire. Il est sous surveillance médicale. Une infirmière arrive pour lui faire une prise de sang.

Infirmière	Bonjour, M. Brown. Comment allez-vous aujourd'hui ?
M. Brown	Comme ci, comme ça. Je n'ai pas très bien dormi la nuit dernière.
Infirmière	Pourquoi n'avez-vous pas appelé l'infirmière de garde ?
M. Brown	Je n'ose pas… Pourriez-vous m'expliquer pourquoi je suis encore sous perfusion ?
Infirmière	Parce que nous devons vous donner des anticoagulants et d'autres médicaments par voie intraveineuse.
M. Brown	Ah, je comprends.
Infirmière	Je dois vous faire une prise de sang maintenant.
M. Brown	Mais vous en avez fait une récemment.
Infirmière	Oui, je sais. Mais comme vous êtes sous anticoagulants nous devons faire un contrôle sanguin régulièrement afin de vérifier si le traitement est efficace. Si l'aiguille vous fait mal, dites-le moi.
M. Brown	Non, ça va. J'y suis habitué maintenant !

Dans la chambre opposée, un infirmier pose une perfusion.

Infirmier	Bonjour, Mme Jones.
Mme Jones	Bonjour.
Infirmier	Je vais vous changer votre perfusion parce qu'elle ne fonctionne pas très bien.
Mme Jones	Qu'est-ce que c'est ?
Infirmier	C'est un garrot. On l'utilise pour mieux voir votre veine. Je vais introduire l'aiguille, ne vous inquiétez pas. Ça peut être un peu douloureux.
Mme Jones	Pourquoi est-ce que suis encore sous perfusion ?
Infirmier	Parce que vous venez d'être opérée. Avez-vous eu des gaz récemment ?
Mme Jones	Non, pas encore.
Infirmier	Alors, votre système digestif est encore un peu lent. Essayez de ne pas trop bouger votre bras pendant que je pose la perfusion.
Mme Jones	Oh, excusez-moi…
Infirmier	Ce n'est pas grave. Je viendrai vous changer la poche toutes les six heures. À plus tard…

Piste 27

Parler de la pression artérielle, de la température et du pouls

Voir p. 82

Médecin	Comment est la pression artérielle de Mme Weeks, aujourd'hui ?
Infirmière	Elle était stable à 15/8 ce matin, mais elle est montée il y a une heure. Peut-être est-ce parce qu'elle a eu de nombreuses visites cet après-midi. Mais tout va bien maintenant. En ce qui concerne sa température, elle est légèrement montée ce matin. Mais elle est stable maintenant. Je l'ai prise il y a une heure, tout est normal. En ce qui concerne M. Jones, son pouls a augmenté. Il est monté jusqu'à 110.
Médecin	Bon. Je vais le voir tout de suite. Mais avant, qu'en est-il de la température de M. Joyce ? Elle est montée à 41 hier soir.
Infirmière	Elle est descendue brusquement ce matin.
Médecin	De combien ?
Infirmière	Elle a baissé de deux degrés mais elle est stable maintenant.

Unit 7

Piste 29

Rassurer le patient

Voir p. 94

Depuis ce matin, M. Brown n'a pas bon moral à cause de ses complications cardiaques. L'infirmière fait de son mieux pour le rassurer et pour qu'il se sente mieux.

Infirmière	Bonjour, M. Brown.
M. Brown	Bonjour.
Infirmière	Comment allez-vous aujourd'hui ?
M. Brown	Pas si bien que ça. Je suis ici depuis deux semaines et je ne vais pas mieux.
Infirmière	Oui, je sais. Mais c'est normal après votre embolie pulmonaire. Maintenant, tout va bien se passer. Vous avez le bon traitement.
M. Brown	Et mon dos m'a fait beaucoup souffrir cette nuit.
Infirmière	Je suis désolée. Mais, vous savez, cela fait longtemps que vous êtes alité.
M. Brown	Et puis… ma famille me manque. Mon fils est reparti en Angleterre la semaine dernière et je me demande maintenant si je reverrai mes petits-enfants.
Infirmière	Ne vous inquiétez pas. C'est vrai que c'est plus difficile d'être malade dans un pays étranger… Mais votre femme vous rend visite tous les jours, n'est-ce pas ?
M. Brown	Oui, c'est vrai. Mais vous savez c'est difficile de lui dire ce que je ressens parfois.
Infirmière	N'hésitez pas à me dire ce qui vous tracasse… Bon, je suis désolée, je dois y aller maintenant, mais je reviendrai cette après-midi et nous en reparlerons. Et n'oubliez pas : l'important c'est de garder le moral.
M. Brown	Merci pour votre aide, à cet après-midi.

Piste 30 Problèmes intestinaux

Voir p. 98

Patiente	Vous savez, docteur, j'ai toujours eu des problèmes intestinaux, mais je ne voulais pas déranger ma famille.
Médecin	Dites-moi, prenez-vous souvent des laxatifs ?
Patiente	Oui, parce que je suis souvent constipée.
Médecin	Mais saviez-vous qu'en fait ils peuvent perturber votre système digestif ?
Patiente	Non, je ne le savais pas.
Médecin	C'est pourquoi vous avez souvent des diarrhées après avoir pris des laxatifs.
Patiente	J'ai des hémorroïdes en plus. Alors, quand c'est très douloureux je prends de l'aspirine.
Médecin	Et dîtes-moi, vos selles sont-elles teintées de sang ?
Patiente	Non.
Médecin	Très bien. Comme je viens de vous le dire, les laxatifs peuvent perturber votre système digestif. Aussi, vous devez manger beaucoup de fruits et boire beaucoup d'eau pour ramollir vos selles. Vous passerez une coloscopie demain.
Patiente	Vous pourriez m'expliquer ce que c'est, s'il vous plaît ?
Médecin	Oui, bien sûr. Nous faisons une coloscopie pour examiner vos intestins avec une coloscope. Mais avant votre examen, vous devez être à jeun. Donc, d'abord vous devrez boire une solution spéciale pour purger votre système digestif. Vous n'avez pas à vous inquiéter.

Unit 8

Piste 35 Conseiller et prévenir

Voir p. 108

Une infirmière donne des conseils à M. Brown et fait de la prévention durant son hospitalisation.

Infirmière	Nous avons besoin de voir différents points afin d'éviter d'autres complications concernant vos problèmes cardiaques et votre diabète.
M. Brown	Très bien, c'est une bonne idée.
Infirmière	Avez-vous envisagé d'arrêter de fumer ?
M. Brown	Oui, bien sûr. Mais j'ai bien peur de ne pas être capable d'arrêter tout seul.
Infirmière	Eh bien, je peux vous proposer une aide pour vous aider.
M. Brown	Pensez-vous qu'il soit possible d'arrêter d'un coup ?
Infirmière	Oui, bien sûr. Vous savez, certaines personnes profitent de leur séjour à l'hôpital pour s'arrêter et elles réussissent. Saviez-vous que votre problème cardiaque était dû au tabac ?
M. Brown	Non, je ne le savais pas.
Infirmière	Et c'est dû également à ce que vous mangez. Vous devriez penser à suivre un régime.
M. Brown	Qu'est-ce que vous me conseillez ?

Infirmière	Tout d'abord, vous allez devoir réduire les graisses animales, le fromage et le beurre, par exemple. Vous devriez faire attention aux viandes grasses, particulièrement les viandes rouges.
M. Brown	Ça va être difficile, j'aime tellement la viande !
Infirmière	Mais vous savez, si vous ne suivez pas votre régime vous aurez des problèmes. Le sucre et les sucreries sont aussi interdits. Mais vous êtes autorisé à prendre des sucrettes.
M. Brown	Et mon poids ?
Infirmière	Vous devez en perdre un peu. Ce serait une bonne idée aussi d'avoir une activité physique, comme marcher par exemple ou faire du vélo.
M. Brown	Merci pour votre aide. Je ferai de mon mieux pour suivre vos conseils.

Piste 37 Au service de cardiologie

Voir p. 112

Infirmière	Vous avez fait un infarctus il y a trois jours. L'électrocardiogramme l'a confirmé. Nous avons dû vous réanimer. Vous devez rester au lit quelques jours.
Patient	Pouvez-vous me dire si c'est la raison pour laquelle j'avais une douleur aiguë à la poitrine et au bras gauche ?
Infirmière	Oui, c'est pour ça. Je viendrai vérifier votre fréquence cardiaque toutes les deux heures et faire un autre électro. Maintenant, voyons voir votre pression artérielle. Euh... 14/8. Je vais l'écrire sur votre feuille de surveillance.
Patient	À quoi ça sert cet appareil, s'il vous plaît ?
Infirmière	Il enregistre votre fréquence cardiaque, ainsi je peux voir si tout va bien. Je vous ai mis deux électrodes sur la poitrine il y a quelques minutes, pour vérifier votre rythme cardiaque.
Patient	Est-ce que je pourrais avoir un autre calmant ? Je souffre encore beaucoup.
Infirmière	Bien sûr. Prenez ce comprimé. Ceci devrait vous aider à vous sentir mieux. Mais avalez-le, ne le laissez pas fondre sous la langue. D'accord ?
Patient	D'accord. Merci.
Infirmière	Je vous en prie.

Unit 9

Éviter les escarres

Voir p. 124

M. Brown est alité depuis trois semaines. Ses talons sont douloureux. L'infirmière lui explique que cela est dû au fait qu'il soit resté longtemps au lit. Elle lui pose des questions pour voir s'il y a d'autres problèmes.

Infirmière Ressentez-vous d'autres douleurs comme des raideurs articulaires ?

M. Brown Non, j'ai seulement mal aux talons.

Infirmière Bien. Êtes-vous constipé en ce moment ?

M. Brown Non, je vais aux toilettes tous les matins.

Infirmière Avez-vous des difficultés pour respirer ?

M. Brown Non. Vous savez, j'ai arrêté de fumer lundi dernier !

Infirmière Félicitations ! Si cela ne vous dérange pas, j'ai d'autres questions. Avez-vous mal quand vous urinez ?

M. Brown Non, pas du tout.

Infirmière Afin d'éviter les escarres vous devez changer de position de temps en temps. Mais si vous avez besoin d'aide pour le faire, dites-le nous. Une aide-soignante viendra vous aider.

M. Brown Et les massages ?

Infirmière Vous aurez un massage une ou deux fois par jour. Je mets un arceau sur le lit pour éviter le poids de la couverture sur vos jambes.

M. Brown Comme c'est gentil. On m'a dit que pour éviter les escarres on utilisait des matelas spéciaux, comme les matelas à coussin d'eau.

Infirmière Oui, c'est exact. Mais le vôtre est un matelas à coussin d'air. N'oubliez pas de boire beaucoup d'eau pour ne pas vous déshydrater.

Pré-médication

Voir p. 129

En chirurgie.

Infirmier Bonjour, Mme White. On va vous opérer dans quelques instants. Je vais vous faire une injection, cela vous aidera à vous détendre avant votre opération. Allongez votre bras. Comment vous sentez-vous ?

Patiente Un peu anxieuse, je dois dire.

Infirmier Ne vous inquiétez pas, tout va bien se passer. On préviendra votre mari quand l'opération sera terminée.

Patiente Vous a-t-il donné le formulaire pour l'autorisation d'opérer ?

Infirmier Oui.

Après l'opération, dans la salle de réveil.

Infirmier Mme White, l'opération s'est bien passée, mais vous devez rester en observation pendant un moment. Je vais vous mettre sous oxygène pendant un moment. Je sais que ce n'est pas très agréable mais essayez de vous détendre. Respirez normalement. C'est ça. Ne vous en faites pas. Vous allez voir votre mari dans un moment.

Unit 10

46 Faire face à un conflit

Voir p. 140

M. Neil, un ami proche de M. Brown, est venu lui rendre visite. Il sort de la chambre et a l'air très en colère.

M. Neil	Je viens de parler avec mon ami et il a très mal au dos. Vous ne pouvez vraiment rien faire pour l'empêcher de souffrir ?
Infirmière	Nous faisons de notre mieux vous savez, mais M. Brown est un peu réservé et il ne nous dit pas quand il a mal.
M. Neil	Ça ne fait rien ! Il est ici depuis trois semaines maintenant et je pense que vous auriez pu faire quelque chose pour le soulager, vous ne croyez pas ?
Infirmière	Malheureusement, M. Brown a eu quelques complications, ce qui n'a pas simplifié les choses.
M. Neil	Et j'aimerais bien avoir des renseignements sur ces complications. Ça m'a l'air difficile d'en obtenir dans cet hôpital !
Infirmière	Malheureusement, je ne peux rien vous dire, c'est à cause du secret professionnel. Cependant, j'aimerais profiter de votre visite pour vous poser des questions à propos de M. Brown. Il se peut que vous ayez des informations le concernant qui pourraient nous être utiles. C'est possible ?
M. Neil	Bien sûr, pas de problème.
Infirmière	Voulez-vous une tasse de café ?
M. Neil	Oui, d'accord.

49 Service de pédiatrie

Voir p. 145

Infirmier	Je suis désolé mais nous devons garder votre bébé pendant quelques jours.
Mère	Pourquoi ?
Infirmier	Il a beaucoup de température à cause d'une otite.
Mère	C'est pour cela qu'il n'arrête pas de se gratter l'oreille gauche ?
Infirmier	Exactement. Dites-moi, êtes-vous à jour de ses vaccins ?
Mère	Oui.
Infirmier	Est-ce qu'il dort d'habitude avec une sucette ?
Mère	Non, mais Brian aime beaucoup son doudou. Je l'ai apporté avec moi. Le voici.
Infirmier	Merci. Quel est son rythme de sommeil ?
Mère	Il fait une petite sieste l'après-midi. Puis-je rester pour l'allaiter ?
Infirmier	Oui, bien sûr et ce sera beaucoup mieux pour lui.

En parlant au bébé.

Infirmier	Ta maman et ton papa vont rentrer à la maison maintenant. Ils ont besoin de se reposer, mais ne t'inquiète pas. Ils reviendront demain et je vais rester avec toi cette nuit. Je vais changer ta couche, elle est toute mouillée. D'accord ? Dodo Brian…

Unit 11

Piste 51 Passer les transmissions

Voir p. 156

Pascale passe les transmissions à Mary. Celle-ci est de garde de midi à 20 heures.

Mary Tu as eu une matinée chargée ?

Pascale Comme d'habitude. J'ai parlé de la sortie de M. Brown avec le chirurgien. Il quittera l'hôpital vendredi prochain. Je n'ai pas eu le temps de lui en parler. Tu peux lui en parler ?

Mary Bien sûr. Je vais lui dire de prendre contact avec une infirmière à domicile. Comme tu sais, il est sous insuline depuis le début de son hospitalisation. Je transmettrai ces informations à sa femme.

Pascale Bien. En ce qui concerne Mme Favre, chambre 14, elle n'est pas aussi bien aujourd'hui qu'hier. Sa température a augmenté. J'ai appelé le Dr Lavau. Il m'a dit qu'il passerait vers six heures.

Mary Et M. Tournier ?

Pascale Le Dr Rainac pense qu'il est nécessaire d'effectuer un certain nombre d'analyses. Il pense à une hépatite B, mais il veut attendre les résultats des analyses pour confirmer ses soupçons. Pourrais-tu t'assurer que les résultats du labo seront prêts quand il arrivera à cinq heures ?

Mary Bien sûr.

Dans la chambre de M. Brown.

Infirmière Bonjour, M. Brown. Alors, vous partez vendredi ?

M. Brown Eh oui. Je voulais m'excuser pour mon ami. Il a été plutôt impoli l'autre jour... Il prend tout tellement au sérieux !

Infirmière Ne vous inquiétez pas, tout s'est arrangé.

M. Brown Merci pour votre aide. Je ne peux pas vous dire à quel point j'ai apprécié votre gentillesse tout au long de mon séjour. Merci beaucoup de m'avoir parlé anglais. Cela m'a vraiment rassuré.

Infirmière Je vous en prie. Bon retour chez vous ! Au revoir !

Piste 53 Chez le gynécologue

Voir p. 160

Médecin À quel âge avez-vous eu vos règles ?

Patiente À quinze ans.

Médecin Quand avez-vous eu vos règles pour la dernière fois ?

Patiente Le 14 août.

Médecin Combien de jours durent-elles ?

Patiente La plupart du temps, cinq ou six jours.

Médecin Sont-elles douloureuses ?

Patiente Surtout le premier jour, mais ensuite ça va.

Médecin	Vos règles sont-elles régulières ?
Patiente	Habituellement, oui.
Médecin	Combien de fois avez-vous été enceinte ?
Patiente	Deux. Mais j'ai fait une fausse couche il y a trois ans.
Médecin	Avez-vous eu des problèmes lors de vos accouchements ?
Patiente	Mon fils est né prématurément à sept mois. Et j'ai eu une césarienne pour ma fille.
Médecin	Merci beaucoup. Maintenant, allongez-vous sur la table d'examen, s'il vous plaît.

Unit 12

Piste 56

Rendre visite à un patient diabétique à domicile

Voir p. 170

M. Brown est maintenant chez lui. L'infirmière à domicile lui parle.

Infirmière	Bonjour, M. Brown. Je suis contente de vous voir de retour chez vous. On m'a dit que vous aviez eu des complications quand vous étiez à l'hôpital ?
M. Brown	Oui, c'est vrai. J'ai passé un moment difficile. En fait, j'ai fait une embolie pulmonaire.
Infirmière	Comment vous sentez-vous maintenant ?
M. Brown	Je me sens beaucoup mieux, bien sûr. Vous savez, j'ai arrêté de fumer et j'ai fermement l'intention de suivre mon régime. À ce propos, j'aurais besoin de quelques conseils. Je n'ai pas très bien saisi ce que je dois faire.
Infirmière	Pas de problème. De toute façon, nous avons tout notre temps. Laissez-moi lire votre ordonnance. Bien, je dois changer votre pansement tous les jours. De plus, je dois vous faire une prise de sang tous les matins.
M. Brown	Et mon diabète ?
Infirmière	Je vais vous montrer comment vérifier votre glycémie et comment vous faire votre injection d'insuline. Les premiers jours, nous le ferons ensemble. Ensuite, vous serez capable de le faire tout seul.
M. Brown	On m'a dit que cétait difficile de le faire seul.
Infirmière	Non, ne vous inquiétez pas. Les nouvelles techniques sont plus simples aujourd'hui. Ce qui est difficile, c'est d'adapter les doses d'insuline à votre glycémie. Mais vous savez, vous vous en sortirez très bien.
M. Brown	À quelle heure viendrez-vous pour ma piqûre demain ?
Infirmière	Je dirais vers 7 heures et demie. Je vous ferai votre pansement également. Je suis sûre que vous allez bientôt aller mieux. À demain.
M. Brown	Au revoir, à demain.

Piste 59 Chez le dermatologue

Voir p. 173

Patient J'ai une éruption de boutons dans le dos et c'est tout rouge.

Médecin Depuis quand ?

Patient Ça a commencé il y a trois jours.

Médecin Avez-vous des démangeaisons ?

Patient Oui, mais je dirais que ça brûle plus que ça ne démange.

Médecin Avez-vous déjà eu une rougeur comme celle-ci ?

Patient Non, c'est la première fois.

Médecin Regardons. Ah, je vois, ça doit être un zona.

Patient C'est grave ?

Médecin Pas trop quand le zona est localisé dans cette région. Mais c'est difficile à soigner. Il vous faudra être patient.

Patient Je vois, d'accord... Ma femme viendra vous voir demain : son eczéma est revenu.

Unit 13

Dialogue entre Mme Wilson et l'infirmière

Voir p. 186

Une infirmière répond aux questions de Mme Wilson concernant l'admission de sa mère en soins palliatifs.

Mme Wilson Être en soins palliatifs, cela signifie-t-il que ma mère va bientôt mourir ?

Infirmière Pas nécessairement. Il est vrai que les soins palliatifs sont au service de beaucoup de personnes qui ont des maladies extrêmement graves ou incurables. Mais, vous savez, certains patients guérissent et n'ont plus besoin d'être en soins palliatifs.

Mme Wilson Vous pourriez me dire ce que signifie exactement soins palliatifs ?

Infirmière Ce sont des soins médicaux spécifiques pour des patients qui ont une maladie grave, comme votre mère. Ce genre de soins concerne avant tout le soulagement des symptômes et du stress occasionné par la maladie. L'équipe soignante est ici pour améliorer la qualité de vie de votre mère et la vôtre également.

Mme Wilson Combien de temps ma mère peut-elle vivre en soins palliatifs ?

Infirmière En général, c'est moins de six mois. Mais votre mère, même avec une espérance de vie de quelques années, peut choisir une approche centrée sur le confort. On lui donnera des conseils sur la douleur et le contrôle de ses symptômes dans le service de consultations.

Mme Wilson Comment savez-vous qu'une personne est prête à aller dans un service de soins palliatifs ?

Infirmière La prise de décision pour entrer en soins palliatifs comprend plusieurs éléments. Dans l'idéal, la décision doit être prise après une discussion avec l'équipe soignante. Certaines questions peuvent nous aider à estimer quand les soins palliatifs deviennent nécessaires.

Mme Wilson De quelles questions s'agit-il ?

Infirmière Par exemple, quelles sont les différentes options possibles pour le traitement ? Que désire la personne malade ? Quelle est la nature et l'évolution de la maladie ?

Mme Wilson Merci beaucoup pour vos réponses.

Infirmière Je vous en prie.

Dialogue entre M. Fear et l'infirmière

Voir p. 192

Une infirmière répond aux questions de M. Fear concernant l'état de son père.

M. Fear Bonjour. Je trouve que mon père dort beaucoup ces derniers jours. Est-ce dû à la morphine ?

Infirmière Oui. Le traitement qu'on lui donne et l'évolution de sa maladie ont tendance à le faire dormir. Cette manifestation clinique provient du ralentissement de son organisme. Nous essayons de soulager ses douleurs de façon à ce qu'il ne s'épuise pas à lutter contre.

M. Fear Et vous pourriez m'expliquer pourquoi vous lui donnez tous ces traitements ?

Infirmière Vous savez, sans eux, sa vie serait insupportable. Jusqu'à présent, il pouvait avaler ses médicaments, mais il ne peut plus le faire. C'est pourquoi nous devons lui donner par voie intraveineuse. Le médecin n'a pas changé le dosage de la morphine et il lui a donné un anxiolytique pour le calmer et le rendre plus détendu.

M. Fear Très bien.

Infirmière Dites-moi, Monsieur Fear, la dernière fois que vous avez rencontré le docteur, vous a-t-il dit pourquoi votre père avait été transféré en soins palliatifs ?

M. Fear Oui. Il m'a dit qu'il était spécialisé dans la prise en charge de la douleur et m'a expliqué ce que signifiaient les soins palliatifs. J'ai compris que le but n'était pas de guérir mais d'améliorer la qualité de vie de mon père et de soulager ses symptômes.

Infirmière C'est cela. Vous avez compris.

M. Fear J'ai également rencontré l'oncologue qui m'a expliqué l'évolution de sa maladie mais je ne pensais pas que mon père était en fin de vie.

Infirmière Comme vous pouvez le voir, il a des difficultés à respirer, des œdèmes et une respiration bruyante. Ce sont des symptômes fréquents en fin de vie.

M. Fear Vous voulez dire qu'il peut mourir à tout moment ?

Infirmière Oui, c'est possible, même s'il est impossible de savoir avec précision quand cela se produira.

M. Fear Je vous remercie pour tout ce que vous faites pour lui et pour moi. Puis-je rester auprès de lui cette nuit ?

Infirmière Bien sûr, nous allons apporter un autre lit. Vous savez, vous pouvez lui parler pour le rassurer, même si votre père semble ne pas réagir à vos mots, il est probable qu'il vous entende.

Rapatriement

Voir p. 197

Une infirmière donne des renseignements à Mme Brown concernant les démarches administratives, les procédures pour le rapatriement du corps et les obsèques de son mari.

Infirmière Tout d'abord, toutes mes condoléances, Mme Brown.

Mme Brown Merci beaucoup. Pourriez-vous me dire ce que je dois faire pour rapatrier le corps de mon mari en Irlande ?

Infirmière Bien sûr. D'abord, vous devez déclarer son décès à la mairie.

Mme Brown Très bien. Dois-je le faire aujourd'hui ?

Infirmière Pas obligatoirement. En fait, vous avez 48 heures. N'oubliez pas d'emporter l'acte de décès.

Mme Brown Pourriez-vous me donner la liste des pompes funèbres, s'il vous plaît ?

Infirmière Oui, la voici. Vous pouvez les appeler ce matin. Ils vous aideront à choisir le cercueil.

Mme Brown Dois-je contacter la compagnie aérienne ?

Infirmière Non, ce n'est pas obligatoire. Les pompes funèbres s'occuperont de réserver le vol. Vous devez leur apporter le passeport et la carte d'identité de votre mari, ainsi que le numéro de téléphone, le nom et l'adresse des pompes funèbres en Irlande.

Mme Brown Combien de jours cela prendra-t-il ?

Infirmière Je ne sais pas exactement. Quelques jours, je suppose. Cela dépend des vols.

Mme Brown En attendant, que va-t-il se passer ?

Infirmière On va transférer le corps à la morgue où il restera jusqu'à ce qu'il soit mis dans un cercueil.

Mme Brown Et en ce qui concerne la crémation ?

Infirmière Vous devez toujours contacter les pompes funèbres. Mais n'oubliez pas de leur dire que votre mari a un pacemaker. Ils doivent l'enlever avant la crémation.

Mme Brown Merci beaucoup pour votre aide.

Infirmière Je vous en prie.

Verbes irréguliers

	Infinitif	Prétérit	Participe passé	Traduction
A	**awake**	awoke	awoken	se réveiller
B	**be**	was/were	been	être
	beat	beat	beaten	battre
	become	became	become	devenir
	begin	began	begun	commencer
	bend	bent	bent	courber
	bet	bet/betted	bet/betted	parier
	bite	bit	bitten	mordre
	bleed	bled	bled	saigner
	blow	blew	blown	souffler
	break	broke	broken	casser
	breed	bred	bred	élever
	bring	brought	brought	apporter
	build	built	built	construire
	burn	burnt/burned	burnt/burned	brûler
	burst	burst	burst	éclater
	buy	bought	bought	acheter
C	**can**	could		pouvoir, être capable
	catch	caught	caught	attraper
	choose	chose	chosen	choisir
	come	came	come	venir
	cost	cost	cost	coûter
	cut	cut	cut	couper
D	**deal**	dealt	dealt	traiter, parler (d'un sujet)
	do	did	done	faire
	draw	drew	drawn	tirer (un trait), dessiner
	dream	dreamt/ dreamed	dreamt/ dreamed	rêver
	drink	drank	drunk	boire
	drive	drove	driven	conduire
E	**eat**	ate	eaten	manger
F	**fall**	fell	fallen	tomber
	feed	fed	fed	donner à manger, nourrir
	feel	felt	felt	sentir, ressentir
	fight	fought	fought	combattre
	find	found	found	trouver
	fly	flew	flown	voler
	forbid	forbade	forbidden	interdire
	forget	forgot	forgotten	oublier
	forgive	forgave	forgiven	pardonner
	foresee	foresaw	foreseen	prévoir
	freeze	froze	frozen	geler

	Infinitif	Prétérit	Participe passé	Traduction
G	**get** **give** **go** **grow**	got gave went grew	got given gone grown	obtenir donner aller pousser, croître, devenir
H	**have** **hear** **hide** **hit** **hold** **hurt**	had heard hid hit held hurt	had heard hidden hit held hurt	avoir, posséder entendre cacher frapper tenir faire mal, blesser
K	**keep** **kneel** **know**	kept knelt knew	kept knelt known	garder, conserver s'agenouiller savoir, connaître
L	**lay** **lead** **lean** **learn** **leave** **lend** **let** **lie** **light** **lose**	laid led leant/leaned learnt/learned left lent let lay lit/lighted lost	laid led leant/leaned learnt/learned left lent let lain lit/lighted lost	poser, mettre (la table) mener, conduire, diriger pencher apprendre laisser, quitter, partir prêter laisser (faire), louer s'allonger, s'étendre allumer, éclairer perdre
M	**make** **may** **mean** **meet** **mistake**	made might meant met mistook	made meant met mistaken	fabriquer, faire pouvoir, avoir le droit/l'autorisation vouloir dire, signifier rencontrer mal comprendre, se tromper
O	**overcome**	overcame	overcome	surmonter
P	**pay** **put**	paid put	paid put	payer mettre, poser
Q	**quit**	quit	quit	arrêter de, abandonner
R	**read** **ride** **ring** **rise** **run**	read rode rang rose ran	read ridden rung risen run	lire monter (à cheval, à bicyclette) sonner, téléphoner se lever (soleil) courir

	Infinitif	Prétérit	Participe passé	Traduction
S	**say**	said	said	dire
	see	saw	seen	voir
	seek	sought	sought	chercher
	sell	sold	sold	vendre
	send	sent	sent	envoyer
	set	set	set	placer
	shake	shook	shaken	secouer, trembler
	shine	shone	shone	briller
	shoot	shot	shot	tirer (coup de feu), abattre
	show	showed	shown/showed	montrer
	shut	shut	shut	fermer
	sing	sang	sung	chanter
	sit	sat	sat	être assis
	sleep	slept	slept	dormir
	slide	slid	slid	glisser
	speak	spoke	spoken	parler
	spell	spelt	spelt	épeler, orthographier
	spend	spent	spent	passer (du temps), dépenser (de l'argent)
	spit	spat	spat	cracher
	spoil	spoilt/spoiled	spoilt/spoiled	gâter
	spread	spread	spread	répandre
	stand	stood	stood	être debout, se tenir debout
	steal	stole	stolen	voler
S	**stick**	stuck	stuck	coller, coincer
	stink	stank	stunk	puer, sentir mauvais
	strike	struck	struck	frapper
	swear	swore	sworn	jurer
	sweep	swept	swept	balayer
	swim	swam	swum	nager
T	**take**	took	taken	prendre
	teach	taught	taught	enseigner
	tear	tore	torn	déchirer
	tell	told	told	dire, raconter
	think	thought	thought	penser
	throw	threw	thrown	jeter
U	**undergo**	underwent	undergone	subir
	understand	understood	understood	comprendre
	undertake	undertook	undertaken	entreprendre
	upset	upset	upset	troubler
W	**wake (up)**	woke	woken	réveiller
	wear	wore	worn	porter (vêtements)
	weep	wept	wept	pleurer
	win	won	won	gagner (jeu)
	withdraw	withdrew	withdrawn	retirer
	write	wrote	written	écrire

Lexiques

Différences orthographiques

GB	US
goitre, fibre	goiter, fiber
oedema, oesophagus	edema, esophagus
diarrhoea	diarrhea
tumour	tumor
anaemia, paediatrician	anemia, pediatrician
leucocyte, ECG	leukocyte, EKG
labelling	labeling
sulphate	sulfate

Français-anglais

A

à moins que : unless
à peine : hardly, barely
à propos : by the way
à quelle distance : how far
à travers : through
abaisser : to lower
abandonner, arrêter de : to give up
absolument : definitely
accélérer : to speed
accompagner : to go with
accomplir : to achieve
accord (être d') : to agree
accord : agreement
accouchement : delivery, childbirth
accru : increased
accueillir : to welcome, to greet
actuellement : currently
adhésion au traitement, observance du traitement : medication adherence
adolescent : teenager
affaibli, détérioré, diminué : impaired
affaiblir : to weaken
affamer : to starve
affirmer : to maintain, to assert
affreux : awful, dreadful
afin de, pour : in order to, to
aggraver (s') : to worsen, to get worse and worse
agrafe : clip
aide-soignante : healthcare assistant, nursing auxiliary, auxiliary nurse (GB), nurse's aid (US)
aiguille : needle
aine : groin
alcoolique : alcoholic
alcooliques anonymes : alcoholics anonymous
alité, cloué au lit, grabattaire : bedridden
allaiter : to breast-feed/to nurse
aller chercher : to fetch
allergique à : allergic to
allonger (s') : to lie down
allumer : to turn on, to switch on
alors que : whereas
améliorer : to improve
amical : friendly
ampoule : vial, phial
amygdale : tonsil
analyse : analysis
anesthésier : to anaesthetize
anesthésiste : anaesthetist
angine : tonsillitis
angine de poitrine : angina pectoris
annuler : to cancel, to call off
antalgique : painkiller
antécédents familiaux : family history
anxiété : anxiety
appareil : device
apparition de cas : outbreak
appeler : to call for, to send for
apprécier : to appreciate, to enjoy
apprendre : to learn
approbation : approval
approfondir : to deepen
arracher (dent) : to pull out
arrêter de, cesser de : to give up, to quit
arrivée : arrival
arriver à, réussir à : to manage
arriver : to arrive, to turn up
arriver (se produire) : to happen, to occur
articulation : joint
ascenseur : lift
asseoir (s') : to sit down
assez : enough, fairly
attacher, lier : to tie, to fasten
attaque : stroke
atteindre : to reach
attelle : splint
attelle gonflable : air splint
attendant (en) : in the meantime
attendre à (s') : to expect
attendre avec impatience : to look forward
attribuer : assign
au-delà de : beyond

au lieu de : instead of
au moins : at least
au régime : on a diet
augmentation : increase, growth
augmenter : to increase, to raise
aussitôt que : as soon as
autoclave : autoclaving
autopsie : post-mortem (examination)
autorisation d'opérer : consent form
autorisé à (être) : to be allowed to
avaler : to swallow
avant-bras : forearm
avérer (s') : to turn out
avertir : to warn
aveugle : blind
avortement : abortion

B

bactérie : a bacterium, bacteria (pl.)
bâiller : to yawn
baisser : to lower, to pull down
balayer : to sweep
bande : strip
bas : low (adj.)
bassin : pelvis (anat.), bedpan
bégayer : to stammer
bénin : benign (tumour GB), (tumor US)
besoin : need
besoin de (avoir) : to need
biberon : feeding bottle, baby's bottle
bibliothèque : library
bien que : although, though
bien s'entendre avec : to get on well with, to get along with
bientôt : soon
bilan de santé : check up
blennorragie : gonorrhoea (GB), gonorrhea(US)
blessé : wounded, injured
blesser, faire mal : to hurt, to injure, to wound
blessure, plaie : wound
boire : to drink
boisson : beverage
bon marché : cheap
bondé : crowded
bonne volonté : good will
bouche : mouth
bouillir : to boil
bouleverser : to distress deeply
bourdonnement : buzzing
bout du doigt : fingertip
bouton : spot
box des urgences : emergency cubicle
brancard : stretcher
brancardier : porter
bras : arm
brassard de tensiomètre : blood pressure cuff
broche : pin
brochure : leaflet
bronzé : suntanned
brosse à dents : toothbrush
brosse : brush
brosser (se) : to brush
bulbe rachidien : medulla
but : goal, purpose, aim

C

cabinet médical : a surgery (GB), an office (US)
cadavre : corpse
cadre de santé : head nurse/senior nurse
caillot : clot
câliner : to cuddle (up)
calmant : painkiller
canine : canine
cannes anglaises : crutches
carnet : log book
carie : cavity
cathéter : catheter
céder : to give in
célibataire : single
cellule : cell
cent, centaine : hundred
cependant : however, yet
cerceau : cradle
cercueil : coffin
cerveau : brain
césarienne : caesarean
chaleur : heat
changer de position : to shift
chauffer : to heat
chercher : to look for, to seek, to search
chef de clinique : registrar

chef de service : senior consultant
chemin : way
chemise de nuit : gown
cher, onéreux : expensive
chercheur : researcher
cheveux : hair (poils = hairs)
cheville : ankle
chiffre : figure
chirurgical : surgical
chirurgie : surgery
chirurgien : surgeon
chlore : chloride
choix : choice
CHU : teaching hospital
cible : target
cibler : to target
cil : eyelash
circulaire, directive : guideline
circulation sanguine : blood stream
ciseaux : scissors
clavicule : clavicle, collarbone
clé : key
cliché radio : X-ray plate
cœur : heart
col de l'utérus : cervix uteri
colère : anger
colère (en) : angry
côlon : colon
colonne vertébrale : spine, backbone
combien de fois : how many times
complètement, entièrement : completely, utterly
compléter, remplir : to fill in (a form)
comportement : behaviour
compréhension : understanding
compresse : swab, compress
comprimé, cachet : tablet
compris (y) : including
compter (sur quelqu'un) : to rely on
concernant, en ce qui concerne : concerning
concubin : concubine
conduire, mener, diriger : to lead
conférence : lecture
confiance : confidence
confiant : confident
conflit : argument, conflict
connaissance : knowledge
conscient : aware
conscient de (être) : to be aware of
conseil(s) : a piece of advice, advice (pl.)
conseiller : to advise
conservateur alimentaire : preservative
consommateur : consumer
consommation : consumption
consommer : to consume
constant, régulier : steady
constipation : constipation
continuer : to go on, to keep on
contrarié/vexé (être) : to be upset
contre : against
contrôle : check
convenable : appropriate
coqueluche : whooping cough
cornée : cornea
corpulent : stout
correctement : properly
côte : rib
côté (à... de) : next to
cou : neck
couche : nappy
couche-culotte : disposable nappy
coude : elbow
couramment : fluently
court : short
couverture sociale : social security cover/ medical insurance
couverture : blanket
cracher : to spit
crâne : skull
crème à raser : shaving cream
crise cardiaque : heart attack
crise d'asthme : asthma attack
critiquer qn pour qch : to blame
croire : to believe
croissance : growth
Croix-Rouge : Red Cross
croyance : belief
cubitus : ulna
cuillère à café : teaspoon
cuillère à soupe : tablespoon
cuir chevelu : scalp
cuisse : thigh
cuvette pour la toilette : washbowl

D

daltonien : colour-blind
de façon à/de sorte que : so that
décennie : decade
décharge : consent form
déchet : waste
déchirure musculaire : pulled muscle
décider (se) : to make up one's mind
décision (prendre une) : to make a decision
déclarer : notify
déclencher : to trigger
décontamination : decontamination
décrire : to describe
déçu : disappointed
déjà : already, ever
déjeuner : lunch
demander (se) : to wonder
démangeaison : rash, itching
déménager : to move
dent(s) : tooth (teeth)
dentier : denture, dental plate
dentifrice : toothpaste
dépêcher (se) : to rush/to hurry
dépendre de : to depend on
dépister, faire subir un test de dépistage : to screen
depuis : since, for
depuis une éternité : for ages
depuis longtemps : for a long time
déranger : to disturb
dernier : last
dès que : as soon as
descendance : offspring
descendre : to go down
détendre (se) : to relax
deuil : bereavement
deux fois : twice
devant : in front of, before
diabète : diabetes
diagnostic : diagnosis
diagnostiquer : to diagnose
diaphragme : diaphragm
diarrhée : diarrhoea (GB), diarrhea (US)
difficile : hard, difficult
dilater : to enlarge
diminuer : to decrease, to cut down, to go down
discuter (avec) : to talk to
disponible : available
docteur : doctor
doigt : finger
dommages : damages
données : data
donneur : donor
dos : back
doucher (se) : to have a shower (GB), to take a shower (US)
douleur : ache, pain
douloureux : aching, painful
drain : drain
drap : sheet
droit (tout) : straight on
droit : right
droitier : right-handed
dur : tough, hard
durée (de vie) : lifespan
durée : duration
durer : to last

E

échantillon : sample, specimen (pour les urines)
écharpe (en) : sling
échec : failure
échelle : ladder
échographie : ultrasound scan
échouer, ne pas arriver à : to fail
écran : screen
effets secondaires : side effects
efficace : effective, efficient
effrayant : scary
égoïste : selfish
élargir : to widen, to broaden
électrode : dot, electrode
éliminer : to eliminate
éloigner (s') : to go away
embryon : embryo
empêcher qn de faire : to prevent someone from doing
empirer : to worsen
emprunter : to borrow
en plus, de plus : moreover
en tenant : holding
enceinte : pregnant

encore : again, still
encourager, inciter : to urge
endormi : asleep, sedated
enfance : childhood
engourdi : numb
engourdissement : numbness
enlever, ôter : to remove, to take off (vêtement)
ennui : boredom
ennuyer (s') : to get bored
ennuyer, tracasser : to bother
ennuyeux : boring
énorme : huge, enormous
enrichissant : enriching, rewarding
enseigner : to teach
ensuite : afterwards
entorse, foulure : sprain
entreprendre : to overtake
entrer : to go in, into, to get in, into
envelopper : to wrap
envers (à l') : upside down
environnement : surrounding
envisager de : to consider
épais : thick
épaule : shoulder
épeler : to spell
EPHAD : home for dependant elderly people
épidémie : epidemic
éponge : sponge
éprouvette : test-tube
épuisant : exhausting
épuisé : exhausted
équilibré : balanced
équipe : team
éradiquer : to wipe out
éruption (cutanée) : skin rash
espérance de vie : life expectancy
espoir : hope
esprit : mind, spirit
essai : trial
essayer : to try
essoufflé : short of breath
essoufflement : shortness of breath, breathlessness
estomac : stomach, tummy
essuyer : wipe
etablissement de soins palliatifs : hospice palliative care
étage : floor
état : condition
été : summer
éteindre : to turn off, to switch off
étendu (être) : to lie
étonnant : amazing
étranger : foreigner
étranger (à l') : abroad
être là, être chez soi : to be in
étroit : narrow
étude, sondage : survey
évaluer : to assess
évanouir (s') : to faint
événement, épisode : event
éviter : to avoid, to prevent
examen : examination, test
excuser (s') : to apologize
exigeant : demanding
expérience : experiment (en labo)
expirer : to breathe out
extérieur (à l') : outside
externe : extern

F

face à (faire) : to cope with, to face
facture : bill
faible, fragile : weak
faim (avoir) : to be hungry
fait (en) : actually
fatigant : tiring
fatigué : tired
fausse couche : miscarriage
faute professionnelle : misconduct
fauteuil roulant : wheelchair
fauteuil : armchair
faux : false
fenêtre : window
fermer (à clé) : to lock
fesse : buttock
feuille de température : temperature chart
feux (circulation) : traffic lights
fiable : reliable
fibre : fibre, roughage
fier : proud
fièvre (avoir de la) : to have a temperature
fil : thread

fille : daughter
finalement : finally, eventually
financer : to fund
fini, terminé : over
fléau, peste : plague
foie : liver
force : strength
forceps : forceps
forme : shape
former (se) : to train
formulaire : form
fort : strong
fou : mad, crazy
fouler (se) : to sprain
fourmillements, picotements : tingling, pins and needles
fournir qch à qn : to provide someone with something
foyer d'épidémie : outbreak
frapper (à la porte) : to knock
fréquence cardiaque : heart-rate
fréquent : common
frissonner : to shiver
front : forehead
frottis : smear test
fumeur (gros) : heavy smoker

G

ganglion : node
gant : glove
garde : shift
garde (de) : on duty
garder le lit : to stay in bed
garrot : tourniquet
gaspiller : to waste
gastro-entérologue : gastroenterologist
gauche : left
gaz (avoir des) : to pass, have wind
gélule : capsule
gencive : gum
gêne : discomfort
genou : knee
gentil : kind, nice
gentillesse : kindness
globe oculaire : eye-ball
glycémie : blood sugar level, glycaemia
gonflement : swelling
gorge : throat
goût : taste
goutte : drop
grâce à : thanks to
graisses : fats
grand et gros : big
grand : tall
graphique : graph
gras, graisse : fat
gratter (se) : scratch
gratuit, libre : free
grave : serious, severe
greffe : graft (de tissu), transplant (d'organe)
grève (en) : on strike
grignoter : to nibble
grippe : flu, influenza
gros : fat
grossesse : pregnancy
grossir : to put on weight
guérir : to cure, to recover, to heal
guérison : cure, recovery
gynéco-obstétrique : ob-gyn
gynécologue : gynaecologist (GB), gynecologist (US)

H

habitué à (être) : to be used to
habituellement, d'habitude : usually
hanche : hip
handicap : disability, handicap
handicapé : disabled, crippled
haut : high
haut, dessus : top
hauteur : height
hémorragie : haemorrhage, bleeding
hémorragie (faire une) : to haemorrhage
hémorroïdes : piles, haemorrhoids
heure (à l') : on time
heures supplémentaires (faire des) : to work overtime
histogramme : bar graph
hors service : out of order
hygiène : hygiene
hypertension artérielle : high blood pressure

I

imagerie par résonance magnétique (IRM) : Magnetic Resonance Imaging (MRI)
imminent : impending
immobile : still
impliquer, signifier : to involve
impliquer (s') : to get involved
impoli, mal élevé : rude
incapable : unable
incisive : incisor
incompréhension : misunderstanding
inconnu : unknown
inconscient : unconscious
inconvénients : drawbacks
indiquer : to direct
inefficace : ineffective
infantile : infantile
infection sexuellement transmissible (IST) : sexually transmitted disease (STD)
infirmière : nurse
infirmière en chef, surveillante générale : matron
infirmière régulatrice : triage nurse
informations, renseignements : information (pl.), a piece of information (sing.)
inoffensive : harmless
insensible : insensitive
insomnie : insomnia
inspirer : to breathe in
insupportable : unbearable
intelligent : clever, intelligent, smart
intense, aigu : sharp, severe, acute
intention de (avoir l') : to intend to, to plan to
interdire : to ban, to forbid
interdit : forbidden
intéresser à (s') : to be interested in
interne : intern
intérieur, interne (adj.) : inner
intervention : procedure
intestins : bowels
intraveineuse : intravenous
inutile : useless
involontaire : involuntary
iris : iris
irréfléchi : thoughtless

J

jamais : never
jambe : leg
jaune d'œuf : egg yolk
jaunisse : jaundice
jetable : disposable
jeter : to throw away
jeun (être à) : to be with an empty stomach, not to eat anything
joue : cheek
jouet : toy
jumeaux : twins
jusqu'à : till
jusqu'à (ce que) : until
jusqu'à présent : so far

K

kinésithérapeute : physiotherapist
kinésithérapie : physiotherapy
kyste : cyst

L

laboratoire, labo : laboratory, lab
laisser tomber : to drop
lait : milk
lame : blade
langue : tongue
large : wide, broad
lavabo : washbasin
laver (se) : to have a wash, to wash
laxatif : laxative
léger : light, slight
léger, bénin : mild
légèrement : slightly
légume : vegetable
lent : slow
lentille : lens
lever : to lift
lever (se) : to get up, to stand up
lèvre : lip
librement : freely
liquide : fluid
lisse : smooth

livre (environ 500 g) : pound
loi : law
loin de : far from
lombalgie, mal de dos : backache
long : long
lunettes : glasses

M

mâcher : to chew
mâchoire inférieure : lower jaw, mandible
mâchoire supérieure : upper jaw, maxilla
maigre : lean, thin
main : hand
maintenir : to maintain
maison de retraite : retirement home
maîtriser : to control
mal : harm
mal de tête : headache
malade : ill, sick
maladie : disease, illness, sickness, complaint
malgré, en dépit de : despite, in spite of
maman : mummy
mamelon : nipple
manger (trop) : to overeat
manière (de cette) : that way
manque de : lack of
manquer (à quelqu'un) : to miss
manquer de : to be lacking in
matelas : mattress
matelas à coussin d'air : air bed
matelas à coussin d'eau : water bed
matériel : equipment
maternité : maternity ward, maternity
mauvais : bad, wrong
médecin : physician, doctor
médecin-chef : consultant
médecin généraliste, traitant : general practitioner (GP)
Médecins sans frontières : Doctors Without Borders
médicament : drug, medication, medicine
médicament sans ordonnance : non prescription drug
meilleur, mieux : better
membre : limb
même si : even if
même, pareil : same
menacer : to threaten
mener, diriger, conduire : to lead
mensonge : lie
menton : chin
mère : mother
mesures : measurements
mieux (faire de son) : to do one's best
mignon : cute
migraine : headache, migraine
mince : slim
mincir : to get slimmer
modèle, schéma : pattern
moelle épinière : spinal cord
moelle osseuse : bone marrow
moindre, moins (le) : the least
moins s'en faire : to take things easier
moins : minus
molaire : molar
mollet : calf
mononucléose : glandular fever
montrer : to show
mordre : to bite
mort (adj.) : dead
mort (n. f.) : death
mortel : deadly
mourir (de) : to die of
moyen : means
moyenne (en) : on average
muet : dumb
mutuelle : mutual (benefit), insurance
myope : short-sighted

N

naissance : birth
nausée : nausea
néanmoins : nevertheless
nécessiter : to require
négligence : carelessness
négligent : careless
nerf : nerve
nervosité : nervousness
nettement : noticeably
nez : nose
nez (qui coule) : running nose
niveau, taux : level

nocif : harmful
nombril : navel, belly button
non-gazeuse : uncarbonated, still
nourrir (au sein) : to breast-feed, to nurse
nourrisson : infant
nouveau-né : newborn
nouvelles : news
noyau : nucleus
nuit (de) : night shift
numération des globules blancs : white blood cell count

O

obèse : obese
obliger : to compel
obscurité : darkness
obstétrique : midwifery
occupé : busy
oculiste : eye-doctor
œdème : oedema
œil : eye
œsophage : gullet, oesophagus
ombilic : umbilicus
omoplate : scapula, shoulder-blade
oncle : uncle
ongle : nail
opérer : to operate on
ordinateur : computer
ordonnance : prescription
oreille : ear
oreiller : pillow
oreillons : mumps
organes génitaux : genitals
Organisation mondiale de la santé (OMS) : World Heath Organization (WHO)
orteil : toe
orthophonie : speech therapy
orthophoniste : speech therapist
os : bone
oser : to dare
ostéopathie : chiropractics
oto-rhino-laryngologiste : ENT specialist
ovaire : ovary

P

pain : bread
pancréas : pancreas
pansement : dressing
paravent : folding screen
parents proches : relatives
paresseux : lazy
parfois : sometimes
parmi : among
partager : to share
passer (du temps) : to spend (time)
passer les transmissions : to pass on reports
patient : patient
patient (atteint du SIDA) : AIDS sufferer (or patient)
patron : boss
paume : palm
paupière : eyelid
peau : skin
peigne : comb
pendant que : while
pénis : penis
penser : to think
perdre : to lose
perfusion (en intraveineuse) : I.V. line
perfusion (être sous) : to be on a drip
perfusion (poser une) : to put up a drip
permettre : to allow
péroné : fibula
personne à prévenir : next of kin
personne âgée : elderly person
personnel (le) : staff
perte : loss
peser : to weigh
petit : small, short
peu (de) : few + pl. , little + sing.
peu probable : unlikely
pharmacie : chemist's, pharmacy
pharmacien : chemist
pharynx : pharynx
phénomènes (un phénomène) : phenomena, (a phenomenon)
pied(s) : foot (feet)
pillule, comprimé : pill
pinces : tweezers

piqûre : injection, sting (abeille)
pipi : wee-wee
pire : worse
place, siège : seat
plaie : wound
plaindre (se) : to complain
plante (du pied) : sole
plaquettes : platelets
plat : dish
plâtre : plaster cast
plein, rempli : full
pleurer : to cry
pleurésie : pleurosis
plomb : lead
plus (de) : moreover
plusieurs : several
poids : weight, burden (sens figuré)
poignet : wrist
poils : hairs (hair = cheveux)
point de suture : stitch
poitrine : chest
pommade : ointment
pompe funèbres : funeral directors
pontage : bypass
postuler : to apply for
pot de chambre (enfant) : potty
poubelle : bin (GB), trash can (US)
pouce : thumb
pouls : pulse
poumon : lung
pousser : to strain, to push
poussière : dust
poux : lice
précédemment : previously
préconiser : to advocate
prélèvement : sample
prendre en compte : take into account
prendre la relève : to take over
prénom : first name, Christian name
préoccupation : concern
presbyte : long-sighted
prescrire : to prescribe
présenter (qn) : to introduce
préservatif : condom
presque : almost, nearly
presque jamais : hardly ever
pressé (être) : to be in a hurry
pression : pressure
prêter : to lend
preuves : evidence
principal, majeur : main
principalement : mainly
prise de sang : blood test
prise de sang (faire) : to take a blood sample
problème : issue, problem
proche (de) : close to
produit laitier : dairy product
professionnels (de la santé) : health professionals
profiter de : to take advantage of
profond : deep
profondeur : depth
projet, plan : scheme
propager (se) : to spread
proportion : ratio
prostate : prostate
protéger : to shelter
prothèse : prosthesis
prothésiste : prosthesist
prouver : to prove
puisque : since
puissant : powerful

Q

quantité : amount
quereller (se) : to quarrel
quiconque : whoever
quoi que ce soit : whatever
quotidien : daily
quotidiennement, tous les jours : daily

R

raccourcir : to shorten
radio : X-ray
rage (de dents) : toothache
raideur : stiffness
raisonnable : sensible
ralentir : to slow down
ramollir : to soften
rapide : fast
rappeler (au tél.) : to call back, to ring back

rappeler (qch à qn) : to remind someone of something
rapport (protégé) : safe sex
rapport, relation : relationship
rare : scarce, rare
rarement : seldom
ras le bol de (avoir) : to be fed up with
raser (se) : to have a shave
rasoir : razor
rassembler : to gather
rate : spleen
réalisation : achievement
réaliser une expérience : to carry out an experiment
réanimation (service) : intensive care
recapuchonner : to recap
recommandation : recommendation
réconfort : comfort
réconforter : to cheer somebody up
reconnaissance : recognition
reconnaître : to acknowledge
réduire : to reduce, to cut down on
refuser, rejeter : to turn down
régime : diet
règle : rule
règles : period(s)
régulièrement : evenly, regularly, steadily
rein : kidney
remarquer : to notice
rembourser : to pay back, to refund
remettre (à plus tard), repousser : to postpone, to put off
remettre en question : to question
remettre, livrer : to deliver
rémission : remission
remplir (formulaire) : to fill in
rendez-vous : appointment
rendre compte (se) : to realize
renforcer : to strengthen
renseigner (se) : to find out, to inquire about
répandu : widespread
repas : meal
répondre : to answer
réponse : answer
repos : rest
reposer (se) : to rest, to have a rest
réserve : supply
résoudre, soulager : to resolve
respiration : breathing
respirer : to breathe
responsable (de) : responsible for
rester : to remain
résultats : findings, results, outcomes
résumer : to sum up, to summarize
retard : delay
retirer : to withdraw
retrait : withdrawal
retraite (prendre sa) : to go on retirement
réunion : meeting
réussir : to succeed in
réussir à un examen : to pass an exam
rhume : a cold
rhume des foins : hay fever
ridé : wrinkled
rideau : curtain
rinçage : rinsing
rincer : to rinse
risque : chance
rond-point : roundabout
roséole : rubeola, roseola
rotule : kneecap, patella
rougeole : measles
rougeur : reddening
rubéole : german measles, rubella
rythme cardiaque : heartbeat

S

sage-femme : midwife
saigner : to bleed
sain, en bonne santé : healthy
salaire : wages, salary
salle d'attente : waiting-room
salle d'opération : operating theatre, operating room
salle de réveil : recovery room
salle de travail : delivery room
SAMU : mobile emergency
sang : blood
sans la peau : skinless
sans surveillance : unattended
santé : health
sauver : to rescue, to save

savon/savonnette : soap
scalpel : scalpel
scanner : CT scan (computed tomography scan)
se défaire : to work loose
sécher : to dry
sécurité : safety
sein : breast
séjour : stay
sélectionner, composer : to dial
selles : stools, faeces
selon, d'après : according to
semaine (dans une) : in a week's time
sensibilité : sensitivity
sensible : sensitive
sentir, ressentir : to feel
seringue : syringe
serré : tight
service (dans le) : on the ward
serviette de toilette : towel
s'excuser de : to apologize
shampoing : shampoo
SIDA : AIDS
sieste : nap
sifflement : wheezing
signes précurseurs, signes avant-coureurs : warning signs
sinon : otherwise
sirop : syrup
sirop pour la toux : cough syrup
soif : thirst
soif (avoir) : to be thirsty
soigner : to cure, to treat, to look after
soins : healthcare
soins à domicile : home medical care
soins en externe : out patient care
soins infirmiers : nursing care
soins intensifs : intensive care
soins palliatifs : palliative care
sol : floor
somnifère : sleeping pill
somnolent : sleepy
sonde : probe
sonner : to ring
sonnette : call button, call bell
sortie : discharge
sortir : to go out
souffrir de : to suffer from
soulager : to relieve
soulagement : relief
soulever : to lift, to raise
sourcil : eyebrow
sourd : deaf
sous-estimé : underestimated
sous-sol : basement
soutenir : to support, to sustain
soutien-gorge : bra
souvenir : memory
spécialiste : specialist, consultant
squelette : skeleton
squelettique : skinny
stable : steady
stade, étape : stage
stage : training
stagiaire : trainee
stérilet : Intra Uterine Device (IUD), coil
stérilisation : sterilization
sternum : breastbone, sternum
subir (une opération, un examen) : to undergo
sucette : dummy
sucre : sugar, glucose
sucrette : (artificial) sweetener
sueur : sweat
suivant : following
suivi (le) : follow-up
suivre : to follow
sujet : topic
supérieur : upper
supplémentaire, complémentaire : further
supportable : moderate
supporter : to bear, to put up with
suppositoire : suppository
sûr, en sécurité : safe
surcharge pondérale (en) : overweight
surexposition : overexposure
surmonter : to overcome
surveillance médicale : medical supervision
surveiller : to look after
survivre : to survive
suturer : to suture, to stitch up

T

table d'examen : couch
tableau : table, chart
tabou : taboo
taches de rousseur : freckles
taille moyenne (de) : medium-sized
tandis que : while
tant que : as long as
tante : aunt
taux : rate
taux (de mortalité) : death rate
téléphoner : to phone, to give a ring, to call
tendance : trend
tension artérielle : blood pressure (BP)
tentative : attempt
tentative de suicide : suicide attempt
tenter : to attempt
terrible, affreux : awful, dreadful
test de dépistage : screening test
testicule : testicle
tête : head
tétine : teat
timide : shy
timidité : shyness
tique : tick
tiroir : drawer
torse, tronc : torso, trunk
tous les combien : how often
tousser : to cough
tout seuls : on their own
toxicomane : drug-addict, drug user
toxicomanie : drug-addiction
trace : tract
trachée : windpipe, trachea
traitement (être sous) : to be on a treatment
tranquillisant : tranquillizer
transmettre (se) : to run in families
transmettre le virus : to pass the virus on
transplantation : transplant
transporter (d'urgence) : to rush
traverser : to go across, to cross
traversin : bedhead
trembler : to shiver
trimestre : term
tronc : trunk
tuer : to kill
tumeur : tumour
tumeur cérébrale cancéreuse : brain cancer
tympan : eardrum

U

uretère : ureter
urètre : urethra
urgences : accident and emergency department, A&E
urine : fluid, urine
urticaire : urticaria
utérus : womb
utile : useful
utiliser : to use
utilité : usefulness

V

vacances : holiday (GB), vacation (US)
vaccin : immunization, vaccination
vagin : vagina
vanter (se) : to boast
varicelle : chicken-pox
varier (de... à) : to range (from... to)
vasodilatateur : vasodilator
venir (chercher qn) : to pick somebody up
ventre : abdomen, belly, tummy
ver : worm
vérifier : to check
vérité : truth
verrue : wart
verser : to pour
vertèbre : vertebra
vésicule biliaire : gall bladder
vessie : bladder
viande : meat
vide : empty
vie (en) : alive
vieillissement : ageing
vision trouble : blurred vision
visites (médecin/inf.) : rounds
volaille : poultry
volonté : will
vomir : to throw up, to vomit, to bring up
vraisemblable (être) : to be likely to
vraisemblance : likelihood
vue : eyesight

Anglais-français

A

A&E: (accident & emergency) les urgences
abdomen: abdomen
abortion: avortement
about: au sujet de/à propos de
about to (be): être sur le point de
abroad: à l'étranger
according to: selon, d'après
account for: prendre en compte, expliquer
ache: douleur
achieve: accomplir, réaliser
aching: douloureux
acknowledge: reconnaître
actually: en fait
acute: aigu/intense
adulthood: âge adulte
adult-onset: commençant à l'âge adulte
advertisement: (une) publicité
advertising: (la) publicité
ad: petite annonce
advice, a piece of advice: conseils, un conseil
advise: conseiller
advocate: préconiser
afterwards: ensuite
again: encore/de nouveau
against: contre
ageing: vieillissement
agree: être d'accord
agreement: accord
AIDS: SIDA
AIDS sufferer patient: patient atteint du SIDA/sidéen
aim: but
aim at: viser
air bed: matelas à coussin d'air
air splint: attelle gonflable
alarm ring: sonnette d'alarme
alcoholic: alcoolique
alive: en vie
allergic to: allergique à
allow: permettre
already: déjà
amazing: étonnant/surprenant
among: parmi
amount: quantité
anaesthetist: anesthésiste
anaesthetize: anesthésier
analysis: analyse
anger: colère
angina pectoris: angine de poitrine
angry: en colère
ankle: cheville
answer: réponse
anxiety: anxiété
apologize: s'excuser
applicant: candidat (à un emploi)
apply for: postuler
appointment: rendez-vous
appropriate: convenable
approval: approbation
argument: dispute
arise: se présenter/survenir (difficulté, question)
arm: bras
arrival: arrivée
as long as: tant que
as soon as: aussitôt que/dès que
asleep: endormi
assess: évaluer
assign: attribuer
asthma attacks: crises d'asthme
at least: au moins
attempt: tenter/tentative
attend: assister régulièrement (à un cours)
audience: public
aunt: tante
available: disponible
average (on): en moyenne
avoid: éviter
aware: conscient
awful: terrible/affreux

B

back: dos
backache: mal au dos/lombalgie
backbone: colonne vertébrale
bacteria/bacterium: bactéries/une bactérie
balanced: équilibré
ban: interdire
bar graph: histogramme
barely: à peine
basement: sous-sol
basis: fondement
be allowed to: être autorisé à/avoir le droit de
be in: être chez soi/être là
be likely to: être susceptible de/vraisemblable
be used to: être habitué à
bear: supporter
bedridden: cloué au lit/alité/grabattaire
behave: se comporter
behaviour: comportement
belief: croyance
believe: croire
belly: ventre
belly button: nombril
benefit: avantager/aider
benign: bénin
bereavement: perte, deuil
better: mieux/meilleur
beverage: boisson
beyond: au-delà
big: grand et gros
bill: facture
bin (GB): poubelle
birth: naissance
bite: mordre
blade: lame
bladder: vessie
blame (somebody of something): critiquer
blanket: couverture
bleed: saigner
blind: aveugle
blood: sang
blood pressure (BP): pression artérielle (PA)
blood pressure cuff: brassard de tensiomètre
blood stream: circulation sanguine
blood sugar level: glycémie
blood test: prise de sang
blood urea nitrogen: urée sanguine
blurred vision: vision trouble
boil: bouillir
bone: os
bone marrow: mœlle osseuse
boredom: ennui
boring: ennuyeux
borrow: emprunter
boss: patron
bother: ennuyer/déranger
bottom: le derrière
bowels: intestins
bra: soutien-gorge
brain: cerveau
brain cancer: tumeur cérébrale cancéreuse
bread: pain
break (have a): faire une pause
breast: sein
breastbone: sternum
breastfeed: nourrir au sein
breath: souffle/respiration/haleine
breathe: respirer
breathlessness: essoufflement
bring: apporter
bring up: vomir
broad: large
broaden: élargir
brush: brosse/brosser (se)
burden: poids
busy: occupé/affairé
buttock: fesse
by the way: à propos
bypass opération: pontage

C

caesarean: césarienne
calf: mollet
call button/call bell: sonnette
call for/send for: appeler
call off/cancel: annuler
canine: canine
capsule: gélule
careless: négligent

carry out an experiment: réaliser/mener une expérience
case report: observation médicale
catheter: cathéter/sonde creuse
cause: causer
cavity: carie
cell: cellule
cervix (uteri): col de l'utérus
chance: risque
cheap: bon marché
check (v.)/check (n.): vérifier/contrôle
checkup: bilan de santé
cheek: joue
cheer somebody up: réconforter
chemist: pharmacien
chemist's: pharmacie
chest: poitrine
chew: mâcher
chicken-pox: varicelle
childbirth: accouchement
childhood: enfance
childish: enfantin
chin: menton
chiropractics: ostéopathie
choice: choix
chronic: chronique
civil servant: fonctionnaire
claim: affirmer/prétendre
clavicle: clavicule
clip: agrafe
close to: près de/proche de
close watch: surveillance
clot: caillot
coffin: cercueil
cold (a): rhume
collarbone: clavicule
cold: froid/rhume
colon: côlon
colour-blind: daltonien
come: venir
come through: survivre
comfort: réconfort
common: fréquent, courant, ordinaire, commun
compel: obliger
complain: se plaindre
complaint: maladie, affection
computed tomography (CT) scan: scanner
computer: ordinateur
concern: préoccupation
condition: état
condom: préservatif
confidence: confiance
confident: confiant
connective tissue: tissu conjonctif
consent form: décharge/autorisation d'opérer
consequently: par conséquent
consider: envisager
constipation: constipation
consultant: médecin-chef
consume: consommer
consumer: consommateur
consumption: consommation
control: maîtriser
cope with: faire face
cornea: cornée
corpse: cadavre
couch: table d'examen
cough: tousser
cough syrup: sirop pour la toux
count: numération
cradle: cerceau
crippled: infirme/estropié
crippling: handicapant
crisis: crise
criterion/criteria: critère/critères
crutches: cannes anglaises
cry: pleurer
CT scan: scanner
cuddle up: câliner/bercer
cure (n.): guérison
cure (v.): guérir
currently: actuellement
curtain: rideau
cut: couper
cut down: diminuer/réduire
cute: mignon
cyst: kyste

D

daily(adj.)/daily(adv.): quotidien/tous les jours, quotidiennement

dairy product: produit laitier
damage: dommages
dare: oser
darkness: obscurité
data: données
daughter: fille
dead: mort
deadly: mortel
deaf: sourd
deal with: s'occuper de/parler de .
death: la mort
death rate: taux de mortalité
decade: décennie
decipher: déchiffrer
decision (make a): (prendre) une décision
decrease: diminuer
deep: profond
deepen: approfondir
definitely: tout à fait/absolument
delay: retard
deliver: accoucher/remettre/livrer
delivery: accouchement
delivery room: salle d'accouchement
demanding: exigeant
depend on: dépendre de
depth: profondeur
describe: décrire
despite: malgré
developing world: pays en voie de développement
device: appareil
diabetes: diabète
diagnose: diagnostiquer
diagnosis: diagnostic (nom)
diagnostic (adj.): diagnostique (adj.)
dial: sélectionner/composer
diaphragm: diaphragme
diarrhoea: diarrhée
die of: mourir de
diet (on a): au régime
differ from: être différent de
direct: indiquer
disability: handicap
disabled: handicapé
disappointed: déçu
disapprove of: désapprouver qch
discharge: sortie
disomfort: gêne, malaise
disease: maladie
dish: plat
disorder: maladie/troubles/désordre
display: afficher
disposable: jetable
disturb: déranger
do one's best: faire de son mieux
Doctors Without Borders: Médecins sans frontières
donour (GB), donor (US): donneur
dot: électrode
drain: drain
dramatically: de manière spectaculaire
drawbacks: inconvénients
drawer: tiroir
dreadful: affreux
dressing: pansement
drink: boire
drill: fraise (dentiste)
drip: perfusion/goutte à goutte
drop (to): chuter/laisser tomber
drop: goutte
drug: médicament
drug user/drug-addict: toxicomane
drug-addiction: toxicomanie
dry: sec
dumb: muet
dummy: sucette/tétine
duplicate: reproduire/dupliquer
duration: durée
dust: poussière
duty (on): de garde

E

ear: oreille
eardrum: tympan
earthquake: tremblement de terre
effective: efficace (traitement)
efficient: efficace (personne)
egg yolk: jaune d'œuf
elbow: coude
elderly person: personne âgée
eliminate: éliminer
embryo: embryon
emergency cubicle: box des urgences
emergency departement: urgences

empty: vide
enjoy: aimer/apprécier
enlarge: dilater
enough: assez
ENT specialist: oto-rhino-laryngologiste
epidemic: épidémie
equipment: matériel
even if: même si
evenly: régulièrement
event: événement/épisode/accident
eventually: finalement
ever: déjà/toujours/jamais
evidence: preuves
exhausted: épuisé
exhausting: épuisant
expect: attendre à (s')
expectations: attentes/espoirs
expensive: cher
experiment: expérience
eye: œil
eye-ball: globe oculaire
eyebrow: sourcil
eye-doctor: oculiste
eyelash: cil
eyelid: paupière
eyesight: vue

F

faeces: selles
fail to: échouer/ne pas arriver à
failure: échec
faint: s'évanouir
false: faux
family history: antécédents familiaux
far from: loin de
fast: rapide
fasten: attacher
fat: gros/gras/graisse
fed up with (be): en avoir assez de
en avoir marre de
fear: crainte, peur
feel: sentir/ressentir
fetch: aller chercher
few (+ pl.): peu de
fibre: fibre
fibula: péroné
figure: chiffre/silhouette
figure out: calculer/trouver
fill in: remplir/compléter (document)
find out: découvrir/se renseigner
findings: résultats
finger: doigt
fingertip: bout du doigt
first name: prénom
floor: étage/sol
flu: grippe
fluently: couramment
fluid: liquide
follow: suivre
following: suivant
follow-up: le suivi
foot/feet: pied/pieds
for a long time: depuis longtemps
forbid: interdire
forbidden: interdit
forearm: avant-bras
forecast: prévision
forceps: forceps
forehead: front
foreigner: étranger
form: formulaire
formerly: précédemment
freckles: tâches de rousseur
free: libre/gratuit
freely: librement
freeze: geler
friendly: amicalement
friendship: amitié
from now on: à partir de maintenant
front of (in): devant
funeral directors: pompes funèbres
further: complémentaire/supplémentaire

G

gall-bladder: vésicule biliaire
gap: fossé/intervalle
gather: rassembler
genitals: organes génitaux
german measles: rubéole
get along/on well: bien s'entendre
get slimmer: mincir
get up: se lever

give a ring: téléphoner
give in: céder
give up: abandonner/cesser de
glandular fever: mononucléose
glasses: lunettes
glove: gant
glucose: sucre
go away: partir/s'éloigner
go down: descendre
go in/into: entrer
go on: continuer
go on retirement: prendre sa retraite
go out: sortir
goal: but
gonorrhea: blennorragie
good at: bon en
good will: bonne volonté
gown: blouse/chemise de nuit
GP: médecin généraliste/traitant
graft: greffe de tissu
graph: graphique
greet: accueillir
groin: aine
grow: croître/augmenter/faire pousser
growth: croissance/augmentation
guideline: directive/circulaire
gullet: œsophage
gum: gencive

H

haemorrhage: hémorragie
hair: cheveux
hairs: poils
hand: main
hand (at): disponible
handicapped (pers.): un handicapé
handsome: beau
hard: difficile/dur
hardly: à peine
hardly ever: presque jamais
hard-working: très travailleur
harm: mal
harmful: nocif
harmless: inoffensif
haste: accélérer, hâter
have a rest: se reposer
have a temperature: avoir de la fièvre
hay fever: rhume des foins
head: tête
head nurse: cadre de santé
headache: migraine/mal de tête
heal: guérir
health: santé
health professionals: professionnels de la santé
healthcare: soins
healthy: sain/en bonne santé
heart: cœur
heart attack: crise cardiaque/infarctus
heartbeat: rythme cardiaque
heart rate: fréquence cardiaque
heat: chaleur/chauffer
height: hauteur
heir: héritier
helpful: serviable/efficace
helpless: désarmé/impuissant
high: haut
high blood pressure: hypertension artérielle
hip: hanche
holding : en tenant
homosexual encounters: rapports homosexuels
hope: espoir/espérer
hospice palliative care: établissement de soins palliatifs
how far: à quelle distance
how long: depuis combien de temps, pendant combien de temps
how many times: combien de fois
how often: tous les combien
however: cependant
HPV: human papillomavirus
huge: énorme
hungry (be): avoir faim
hundred: cent/centaine
hurt: blesser/faire mal
hygiene: hygiène
hypothesis: hypothèse

I

I.V. line: perfusion intraveineuse
ill: malade

illness: maladie
immunization: vaccin
impaired: affaibli/détérioré/diminué
impending: imminent
improve: améliorer
inch: pouce (environ 2,5 cm)
incisor: incisive
including: y compris
income: revenu
increase: augmenter/augmentation
increased: accru
ineffective: inefficace
infant: nourrisson
influenza/the flu: la grippe
information: renseignements
injection: piqûre
injure: blesser
inner: intérieur/interne
insensitive: insensible
insomnia: insomnie
instead of: au lieu de
insurance: mutuelle/assurance/garantie
intake: prise
intensive (care): soins intensifs/réanimation
interested in (be): s'intéresser à
Intra uterine device (IUD): stérilet
introduce: présenter (qn)
involve: impliquer, signifier
involved (be): s'impliquer
involvement: implication
iris: iris
irrelevant: hors de propos
issue: problème
itching: démangeaison

J

jaundice: jaunisse
jaw: mâchoire
joint: articulation
jump: sauter/bondir

K

keep in bed: garder le lit
keep on: continuer
key: clé
kidney: rein
kill: tuer
kind: gentil
kindness: gentillesse
knee: genou
kneecap: rotule
knife: couteau
knock: frapper (à la porte)
knowledge: connaissance

L

laboratory: laboratoire
lab: labo
lack of: manque
lame: estropié
last: durer/dernier
late: en retard/tard
laugh at: se moquer
law: loi
laxative: laxatif
layer: couche
laziness: paresse
lazy: paresseux
lead: conduire/mener/diriger
leaflet: brochure
lean: maigre
learn: apprendre
least: le moindre/le moins
left: gauche
leg: jambe
lend: prêter
length: longueur
lengthen: allonger
lens: lentille
level: niveau/taux
library: bibliothèque
lice/louse: pou/poux
lie: être étendu/mentir/mensonge
lie down: s'allonger
life expectancy: espérance de vie
life-threatening: esxtrêmement grave
lifespan: durée de vie
lift: ascenseur/soulever
light: léger
likelihood: vraisemblance
limb: membre

link to: associer à/lier à
lip: lèvre
liver: foie
lock: fermer à clé
log book: carnet
long: long
long for: se languir
long-sighted: presbyte
look after: surveiller
look forward to: attendre avec impatience
lose: perdre
loss: perte
low: bas
lower: abaisser
lower jaw: mâchoire inférieure
lung: poumon
lymph-node: ganglion lymphatique

M

mad: fou
Magnetic Resonance Imaging (MRI): Imagerie par résonance magnétique (IRM)
main: principal/majeur
mainly: surtout/principalement
maintain: maintenir
make up one's mind: décider (se)
manage: arriver à/gérer
management: prise en charge
mandible: mâchoire inférieure
marrow: moelle
maternity ward: maternité
matron: infirmière en chef/surveillante générale
maxilla: mâchoire supérieure
mattress: matelas
meal: repas
mean: moyen
meantime (in the): en attendant
measles: rougeole
measurements: mesures
meat: viande
medication: traitement
medication adherence: adhésion au traitement/observance du traitement
medicine: médecine/médicament
medium-sized: de taille moyenne
medulla: bulbe rachidien/moelle
meeting: réunion
memory: souvenir
metacarpal: métacarpien
midwife: sage femme
midwifery: obstétrique
mild: léger/bénin
milk: lait
mind: esprit
minus: moins
miscarriage: fausse couche
misconduct: faute professionnelle
misunderstanding: incompréhension
miss: manquer (à quelqu'un)
moderate: supportable
molar: molaire
moreover: de plus/en plus
mother: mère
motherhood: maternité
mouth: bouche
move: déménager
mumps: oreillons

N

nail: ongle
nap: sieste
narrow: étroit
nausea: nausée
navel: nombril
nearly: presque
neck: cou
need: avoir besoin/besoin
needle: aiguille
nerve: nerf
nevertheless: néanmoins
nervousness: nervosité
newborn: nouveau-né
news: nouvelles
next of kin: parent proche (personne à prévenir)
next to: près de
nibble: grignoter
nicely: gentiment/doucement
night shift: équipe de nuit

nipple: mamelon
node: ganglion
non prescription drugs: médicament sans ordonnance
nose: nez
notice: remarquer
noticeably: nettement
notify: déclarer
numb: engourdi
numbness: engourdissement
nurse: infirmière
nurse: allaiter
nurse's aid (US): aide-soignante
nursing care: soins infirmiers

O

obese: obèse
Ob-Gyn: gynéco-obstétrique
obvious: évident
obviously: de façon évidente/évidemment
occupational: professionnel
occur: arriver/se produire
oedema: œdème
oesophagus: œsophage
offspring: descendance/progéniture
ointment: pommade
on their own: tout seuls
operate on: opérer
operating theatre/room: salle d'opération
order to (in): dans le but de/pour/afin de
otherwise: sinon
out of order: en panne
outcome: résultat
outpatient care: soins en externe
outbreak: foyer d'épidémie
outer: extérieur/externe
ovary: ovaire
over: fini/terminé
overcome: surmonter
overcrowded: bondé
overeat: trop manger
overweight: surcharge pondérale

P

pain: douleur
painful: douloureux
painkiller: antalgique/calmant
palliative care: soins palliatifs
palm: paume
pancreas: pancréas
paradoxically: paradoxalement
pass an exam: réussir un examen
pass on reports: passer les transmissions
pass the virus on: transmettre le virus
patella: rotule
pattern: modèle/schéma
pay back: rembourser
pelvis: bassin (anat.)
perform: réaliser/faire
period(s): règles
pertussis: coqueluche
pharynx: pharynx
phenomena (a phenomenum): phénomènes (un phénomène)
phial: ampoule
physician: médecin
physiotherapist: kinésithérapeute
physiotherapy: kinésithérapie
pick someone up: venir chercher qn
piles: hémorroïdes
pill: pilule/comprimé
pin: broche
pins and needles: picotements et fourmillements
plague: fléau/peste
plan to: avoir l'intention de
platelet: plaquette
plaster cast: plâtre
pleurosis: pleurésie
plump: dodu
post-mortem examination: autopsie
postpone: différer/remettre à plus tard
poultry: volaille
pound: livre (environ 500 g)
potty: pot de chambre (enfant)
pour: verser
powerful: puissant
pregnancy: grossesse
prescribe: prescrire
prescription: ordonnance
preservative: conservateur alimentaire
pressure: pression
prevent somebody from: empêcher qn de

probe: sonde
procedure: examen/intervention
pro-life activist: opposant à l'avortement
promote: promouvoir
properly: correctement/convenablement
prosthesis: prothèse
prosthetist: prothésiste
protect from: protéger de
proud: fier
prove: prouver
provide somebody with something: fournir qch à qn
provided: à condition que
public health officials: autorités sanitaires
pull out: arracher
pulled muscle: déchirement musculaire
pupil: pupille
purpose: but
put off: remettre à plus tard
put on weight: grossir
put up (a drip): poser une perfusion
put up with: tolérer/supporter

Q

quarrel: disputer (se)
question: remettre en question
quite: assez/très

R

raise: soulever (un problème), augmenter
range from… to: varier de… à
rash: démangeaison/rougeur/éruption/ plaques d'urticaire
rate: taux
ratio: proportion
razor: rasoir
reach: atteindre
realize: se rendre compte
recap: recapuchonner
recognition: reconnaissance
recommendation: recommandation
recover: guérir
recovery: guérison
recovery room: salle de réveil
Red Cross: Croix-Rouge
reddening: rougeur
reduce: réduire
refer somebody to: adresser qn à
refund: rembourser
regarding: concernant/en ce qui concerne
registrar (senior registrar): chef de clinique
regulations: règlements
relationships: relations/ rapports
relatives: parents/proches
reliable: fiable
relief: soulagement
relieve: soulager
reluctant: réticent
rely on: compter sur quelqu'un
remain: rester
remark: faire remarquer
remind somebody of something: rappeler qch à qn
remove: enlever
replacement: remplacement
reproach somebody for something: reprocher qch à qn
require: nécessiter
rescue: sauver
researcher: chercheur
resolve : résoudre, soulager
responsible for: responsable de
rest (have a): repos/se reposer
retirement home: maison de retraite
results: résultats
rewarding: enrichissant
rhythm: rythme
rib: côte
right: droit
right-handed: droitier
ring: sonner
ring back: rappeler au téléphone
rinse: rincer
rinsing: rinçage
rise: augmenter/s'élever
roughage: fibre
roughly: en gros/à peu près
roundabout: rond-point
rounds: visites
rubella: rubéole
rubeola: roséole
rule: règle

run in families: se transmettre/être héréditaire
running nose: nez qui coule
rush: transporter d'urgence/se dépêcher

S

safe: sûr/en sécurité/coffre
safe sex: rapport protégé
safety: sécurité
salary: salaire
sale: vente
same as (the): (le) même que
sample: échantillon/prélèvement
save: sauver
scale: échelle
scalp: cuir chevelu
scapula: omoplate
scar: cicatrice
scary : effrayant
schedule: programme
scheme: projet/programme
scissors: ciseaux
scratch: se gratter
screen(v.)/screen(n.): dépister/écran
screen folder: paravent
screening test: test de dépistage
seat: place/siège
sedated: endormi
seek: chercher
seldom: rarement
selfish: égoïste
senior consultant: chef de service
sensible: raisonnable/sensé
sensitive: sensible
sensitivity: sensibilité
serve: être au service de
several: plusieurs
sexually transmitted disease (STD): infection sexuellement transmissible (IST)
shampoo: shampoing
shape: forme
share: partager
sharp: pointu/tranchant/aigu
shaving cream: crème à raser
sheet: drap
shift: garde
shift: changer de position
shingles: zona
shiver: frissonner/trembler
short: court
short of breath: essoufflé
shorten: raccourcir
shortness of breath: essoufflement
short-sighted: myope
should: vous devriez, il faudrait que…
shoulder: épaule
shoulder-blade: omoplate
show: montrer
shy: timide
shyness: timidité
sick: malade
sickness: maladie
side effects: effets secondaires
significant: important/significatif
silly: idiot
since: depuis/puisque
single: célibataire/unique
skeleton: squelette
skin: peau
skin rash: éruption cutanée
skinless: sans la peau
skinny: squelettique
skull: crâne
sleeping pill: somnifère
sleepy: somnolent/endormi
slight: léger
slightly: légèrement
slim: mince
sling: écharpe (en)
slow: lent/ralentir
slowness: lenteur
small/short: petit
smallpox: variole
smart: intelligent
smear test: frottis
smoker: fumeur
soap: savon/savonnette
so far: jusqu'ici
soften: ramollir
so that: de façon à ce que/de sorte que
sole: plante du pied
sometimes: quelquefois/parfois
soon: bientôt
span: durée (de vie)

spare: épargner
specialist: spécialiste
specimen: échantillon pour urine
speech therapist: orthophoniste
speech therapy: orthophonie
speed: accélérer
spell: épeler
spend: passer (du temps)/dépenser (de l'argent)
spinal cord: mœlle épinière
spine: colonne vertébrale
spit: cracher
spleen: rate
splint: attelle
split: séparer (se)
sponge: éponge
spot: bouton
sprain(v.)/sprain(n.): fouler (se)/entorse/foulure
spread: propager (se)
staff: personnel (le)
stage: stade/étape
stammer: bégayer
stamp: timbre
stand: se tenir debout
stand for: représenter
starve: affamer/mourir de faim
stay: séjour
steady: constant/régulier
sterilization: stérilisation
stiffness: raideur
still: immobile
stitch: point
stomach: estomac
stools: selles
stout: corpulent
straight on: tout droit
strain: pousser
strength: force
strengthen: renforcer
stretcher: brancard
strike: frapper
strike (on): en grève
strip: arracher/dénuder/bande
stroke: attaque
strong: fort
succeed in: réussir à
such: tel
suffer from: souffrir de
sugar: sucre
suicide attempt: tentative de suicide
summarize: résumer
sunburnt: brûlé (au soleil)
suntan lotion: crème solaire
suntanned: bronzé
supply: réserve
supply somebody with: fournir
support: soutenir
suppository: suppositoire
surge in: poussée/augmentation de
surgeon: chirurgien
surgery (a): chirurgie/cabinet médical
surgical: chirurgical
surrounding: environnement
survey: étude/sondage
suture: suturer
swallow: avaler
sweat: sueur
sweep: balayer
sweetener (artificial): sucrette
sweets: bonbons
swelling: gonflement
switch off: éteindre
syringe: seringue

T

table: tableau
tablespoon: cuillère à soupe
tablet: comprimé/cachet
taboo: tabou
take advantage of: profiter de
take into account: prendre en compte
take somebody seriously: prendre quelqu'un au sérieux
take over: prendre la relève
take things easier: moins s'en faire
talk to: parler à/discuter
tall: grand
tan: bronzage
target: cible/cibler
taste: goût
teach: enseigner/apprendre
teaching hospital: centre hospitalier universitaire (CHU)

team: équipe
teaspoon: cuillère à café
teat: tétine
teenager: adolescent
temperature chart: feuille de température
tender: sensible
term: trimestre
testicle: testicule
test-tube: éprouvette
thanks to: grâce à
thick: épais
thigh: cuisse
thin: maigre
thirst: soif
thirsty (be): avoir soif
though: bien que
thought: pensée
thread: fil
threat: menace
threaten: menacer
throat: gorge
through: à travers/par
throw up: vomir
thumb: pouce
tick: tique
tie (up): attacher/lier
tight: serré
till: jusqu'à
tingling: fourmillement/picotement
tired: fatigué
tiring: fatigant
toe: doigt de pied/orteil
tongue: langue
tonsil: amygdale
tonsillitis: amygdalite, angine
tooth (teeth): dent(s)
toothbrush: brosse à dent
toothache: mal de dent
toothpaste: dentifrice
top: haut/dessus
topic: sujet
tough: dur/rude
tourniquet: garrot
toy: jouet
tract: trace
train: se former/faire une formation, un stage
trainee: stagiaire
training: stage
transplant: transplantation
trash can (US): poubelle
travel: voyager
treat: soigner
treatment (on a): sous traitement
trend(v.)/trend (n.): avoir tendance à/tendance
triage nurse: infirmière régulatrice
trial: essai
trigger: déclencher
true: vrai
trunk: torse/tronc
truth: vérité
try: essayer
tummy: ventre
turn down: refuser/rejeter
turn off: éteindre
turn on: allumer
turn out: s'avérer
turn up: arriver
tweezers: pinces
twice: deux fois
twins: jumeaux

U

ugly: laid
ulna: cubitus
ultrasound scan: échographie
unable: incapable
unattended: sans surveillance
unbearable: insupportable
uncarbonated: non gazeux
uncle: oncle
unconscious: inconscient
underestimated: sous estimé
undergo: subir (une opération)
understanding: compréhension
undertake: entreprendre
unknown: inconnu
unless: à moins que
unlikely: peu probable
until: jusqu'à ce que
upper: supérieur
upper jaw: mâchoire supérieure
upset: bouleverser
upset (to be): être contrarié/vexé

upside down: à l'envers
ureter: uretère
urethra: urètre
urge: encourager/inciter
urticaria: urticaire
use: utiliser
used to (be): être habitué à
useful: utile
usefulness: utilité
useless: inutile
usually: d'habitude/habituellement
utterly: complètement

V

vaccination: vaccin
vagina: vagin
vasodilator: vasodilatateur
vegetable: légume
vertebra: vertèbre
vertebral column: colonne vertébrale
vessel: vaisseau
vial : ampoule

W

water bed: lit à coussin d'eau
waiting-room: salle d'attente
wall: mur
ward (on the): dans le service
warn: avertir
warning signs: signes précurseurs/signes avant-coureurs
wart: verrue
wash (have a): se laver
washbasin: lavabo
washbowl: cuvette pour la toilette
washcloth: gant de toilette
waste: déchet/gaspiller
way: chemin/façon/manière
weak: faible/chétif
weaken: affaiblir
weakness: faiblesse
wee-wee: pipi
week's time (in a): dans une semaine
weigh: peser
weight: poids
well-known: très connu
whatever: quel que soit/quoique ce soit
wheelchair: fauteuil roulant
wheezing: sifflement
whereas: alors que/tandis que
whether: si
while: pendant que
white blood cell count: numération des globules blancs
whoever: quiconque
whooping cough: coqueluche
wide: large
wide open: grand ouvert
widen: élargir
widespread: répandu
will: volonté
wind: gaz/vent
windpipe: trachée
window: fenêtre
wipe: essuyer
wipe out: éradiquer
withdraw: retirer
womb: utérus
wonder: se demander
work loose: se défaire
work overtime: faire des heures supplémentaires
World Health Organization (WHO): Organisation mondiale de la santé (OMS)
worse: pire
worsen: empirer
worst (the): le pire
wound: blesser/blessure
wounded: blessé
wrap: envelopper
wrinkled: ridé
wrist: poignet

X - Y

X-ray: radio
X-ray plate: cliché radio

yawn: bâiller
yawning: bâillement
yet: déjà/cependant
yet (not): pas encore/toujours pas

PEFC PEFC/30-32-821

Achevé d'imprimer en avril 2021
par Wilco aux Pays-Bas
Dépôt légal: mai 2021
N° éditeur MAGSI20200121